D0593439

Survival Guide

Anatomy
and Physiology

Survival Guide

FOR

Anatomy
and Physiology

Tips, Techniques
and Shortcuts

FOR

Learning about the Structure and Function
of the Human Body
with Style, Ease, and Good Humor

KEVIN T. PATTON

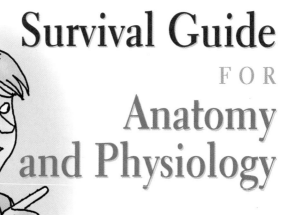

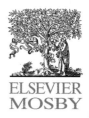

ELSEVIER
MOSBY

MOSBY
ELSEVIER
11830 Westline Industrial Drive
St. Louis, Missouri 63146

Survival Guide for Anatomy & Physiology   ISBN-13:   978-0-323-04330-4
                                             ISBN-10:   0-323-04330-5

Notice
Neither the Publisher nor the authors assume any responsibility for any loss or injury and/or damage to persons or property arising out of or related to any use of the material contained in this book. It is the responsibility of the treating practitioner, relying on independent expertise and knowledge of the patient, to determine the best treatment and method of application for the patient.

The Publisher

ISBN-13: 978-0-323-04330-4
ISBN-10: 0-323-04330-5

Executive Editor: Tom Wilhelm
Managing Editor: Jeff Downing
Publishing Services Manager: Gayle May
Cover Designer: Mark Oberkrom

Working together to grow
libraries in developing countries
www.elsevier.com | www.bookaid.org | www.sabre.org

ELSEVIER   BOOK AID International   Sabre Foundation

Printed in the United States of America

Last digit is the print number: 9 8 7 6 5 4 3 2 1

About this Book

H i! I'm Kevin Patton, the author of this survival guide. I've enjoyed several decades of studying human anatomy and physiology—and also studying how to study this subject. Besides taking courses in "A & P" at the high school, college, and graduate levels, I have also taught it at all three levels. I still study A & P informally as I work on my textbooks and as I prepare the classes I teach at a community college and university. I also study A & P several times each year at formal workshops and seminars. During this time, I've come to appreciate that the major keys to success in any A & P course are style and attitude. This book will help you with both by giving you some simple and clear tips on how A & P can be easily and quickly mastered.

This survival guide can be used easily in any A & P course with any textbook. In fact, you can use much of it in your other courses!

This survival guide for anatomy and physiology students begins with a quick and easy overview of some of the strategies my students and I have used to make our studies more productive—and therefore more fun and less time consuming. Scattered throughout this first part, I've included several boxes conspicuously titled "Hints" and other special boxed sections that cover topics of interest to many students. For example, a special box for returning or nontraditional students is offered, a box on learners with special needs, a box on learning in the laboratory, and a box for using the computer to help study A & P. You'll also find sidebars that highlight some of the more important points in this guide.

If you find that a thoughtful look at how you study has a positive effect on the efficiency of your studying—and I'm sure that it will—then I encourage you to talk to your professor, college librarian, or a learning center specialist to find out more ways to help yourself learn A & P and other subjects.

The second part of the book is a handy compilation of diagrams, charts, and tables that serve as quick "field guides." This collection of resources will help you as you study, in the lab, and even later in clinical or applied situations because they contain much of the essential information needed to understand the human body's structure and function. The diagrams are like pocket maps to the body, quickly getting you on the right road when you're lost. The charts and tables summarize facts in a way that will help you organize your own thinking about important concepts—and they will help you remember the details when they slip your mind.

The second part also includes a scattering of analogies and models that you will find helpful in learning some of the trickier concepts of A & P.

I'm using the analogy of survival in a wilderness throughout this book for at least two reasons. First, beginning students often do feel overwhelmed in an unfamiliar territory. Secondly, it is a good analogy—many of the skills you might use to survive in the wilderness have their counterparts in coping with your A & P course. Importantly, as we shall learn, analogies make learning easier.

I'd love to get any feedback on this guide that you'd like to share with me—good or bad; or perhaps you'd like to share some learning secrets you've discovered. Contact me at the following web site address: http://www.lionden.com

Kevin Patton
Weldon Spring, Missouri

HINT

☑ Read this guide before you begin your A&P course—or as soon after starting it as you can.

☑ Review the different survival strategies in this guide from time to time throughout the rest of your course.

Dedication

This book is dedicated (in no particular order) to Andrew, Aileen, Luke Baraka, Jenny-tamu, Tom, Pat, Rick, Will, Mallory, Jeanne, Max, Sammee, David and Sue, Gary and Emogene, Gail, Sally, Robyn, Cathy, Dan, Heather, Corkey the Wonder Dog, the members and staff of HAPS, Jules Jacot, Tom, Jeff, Gordon and Rosie, Carol, John M., Pat (a different Pat than the one mentioned previously), Michael, several Mikes, Audrey, Barb, the Cindies, fellow members of the Irish Diaspora, Laura, Ron Giedinghagen, Clyde, Jill, Ed, the SCC crowd, Jacqueline, Karen, Timba and Dante (wherever they are), Thomas Jefferson, Jessica, The Flying Wallendas, Ivor (David), TC Westfall, Monty Python, Roger Tory Peterson, Ann, Zoe, Mary Ann, Debbie, Gene, Stacey, John B., Tracy, Bob, Robert Heinlein, Nurse Kelly, Yvonne, Gracie Allen, Alfred Court, NABT, Hal, Pastor Dena, The Royal Liechtenstein Circus, Takeshi, United Republic of Tanzania, Mandy, Marlin and Carol Perkins, Sister Virginia, Alpha Calhoun, the Empress Cris, Jack and Mike, Father Mulligan, Professor Keller, Paris (the city), Aunt Al, Jerry, Loretta, Leonardo Da Vinci, Gunther, Sarah and Michael, Flora, Wayne Franzen, Stormy, St. Louis Zoo and WBS alumni, Mary Ellen McDonald, Ana Mary, Gregor Mendel, Jim, Daniel, Miss Jones, Winnie, C.V. Mosby and Catherine Anthony, the LRC staff, the Butz family, DB, Ira, Peter, H.S.H. Prince Rainier and the Monte Carlo Circus Festival, Marjorie, Andreas Vesalius, April, Caoimh'n, Stefanie, Steve, Jean, Mr. Bean, Michelle, SLU Pharm/Phys, Fr. John, CFA, Mysté, Greenway Network, Mahatma Gandhi, the Chieftains, Saitoti, Rhonda, Dora, Pam, Bill-Jim, Lucia, Margaret, Dayton (not the city), Ned Devine, W.B. Yeats, Bill, Reneé, the Kaigai family, John Dominic, Mary Alice, Chaya, and Julie Bowen.

Contents

Survival Guide

FOR

Anatomy
and Physiology

PART 1

Introduction to the Survival Skills

A s you begin a new course, you may feel as though you're wandering in a wilderness where the ideas are strange, the language unique, and the terrain unfamiliar. In other words, you feel a little lost. *Have no fear!* This guide provides a set of survival skills to help you in your trek through the strange and wondrous world of human anatomy and physiology (A&P).

Take the time to have a good look at the skills outlined in the following pages. Some you will find useful; others may not suit your style. The important thing is to give some thought to your style of learning and your attitude in this great adventure that you're starting. I guarantee that any time given to working on your approach to studying will be returned to you at least tenfold!

Choose those strategies that *work for you*—then *use them!*

HINT

☑ The inside front cover lists the ten Survival Tips. *Each time* you start a new topic, briefly check the list of Survival Tips to make sure you're not forgetting something.

Have a Winning Attitude

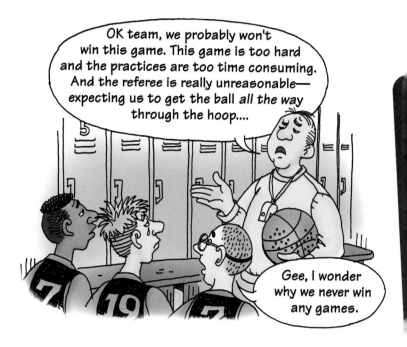

In the introduction to this guide, I stated that the major keys to success in any A&P course are *style* and *attitude*. I'll tell you more than you probably want to know about style in Survival Skill 2. For now, let's concentrate on attitude.

You may have heard a hundred times (perhaps it seems like a million) that a winning attitude is an important key to success. There really is a lot of truth to this however, especially when it comes to learning. Before I started teaching, I was a lion tamer in the circus (no kidding!); before that I trained marine mammals at a zoo. In both situations I found that my animals learned new behaviors really fast and really well *if they were having fun* or if they were *highly motivated.* If they were *both* having fun *and* highly motivated—the results were incredible!

With both my African lions and my sea lions, I was the one setting the learning goals—so it was up to me to set the attitude. I only asked my animals to do things that they found to be fun (by watching them play on their own) and by giving them food rewards and praise (lions, by the way, will do almost anything for a hug and a kind word). In your situation, however, setting the attitude is *up to you.* It's as simple as deciding to have a positive, winning attitude. As goofy as it might sound, just telling yourself you're successful in your A&P course is enough to dramatically improve your chances of success. It's just like the cases of patients who refuse to give in to their injuries or illnesses and jump into therapy with gusto—they're always the ones who exceed all normal expectations of recovery.

If you consistently resist and counteract negative thinking (such as "I'll never be able to understand this concept"), you'll actually have an even better chance at shining success in A&P.

One place you can always count on someone helping you getting and maintaining a winning attitude is your professor's office. Like a good animal trainer—or a winning coach—your professor will always take the time to talk to you about your studies and help you keep the proper attitude. Even professors that might seem a little intimidating that first day in class *always* turn out to be caring, willing helpers in your struggles with A&P. As President Emeritus of the Human Anatomy and Physiology Society (HAPS), I've gotten to know literally thousands of A&P teachers across North America and beyond. All of those people *love* A&P and *love* teaching it. They really enjoy helping people like you find success in a subject that is very exciting for them. When that enthusiasm rubs off—and it will—you'll be that much closer to reaching your goal.

Your professor will always take the time to talk to you about your studies and help you keep the proper attitude.

So what about the *fun* and the *motivation?* Let's start with the fun (a motto to live by). Your instructor's enthusiasm (if you open yourself up to it) will get you started on the road to having fun. Then, try to get into a study group. I'll talk more about the learning value of this strategy later in Survival Skill 7, but right now let's concentrate on the fun. Getting together with other A&P students for study sessions can be fun. Take turns hosting sessions by rotating who chooses times and places. Perhaps bring snacks or go out for snacks as a group. Make it as much a social gathering as an academic endeavor.

I'm not suggesting that you go out and party on the pretext that you're studying. I'm saying instead that studying as a group can be fun if you decide to make it fun. Laugh, joke around, gossip, whatever — but stay at least loosely focused on learning your topic. Don't end the "party" until you've reached the learning goal you've set for yourselves. Then, as you get to know one another better, you may want to try a social outing or two. Getting to know people outside the classroom or study session often makes your academic partnerships more effective.

Another way to make A&P fun is to involve other people that aren't even in your A&P class. If you have friends or family that might like to share some of the time you're spending with your A&P studies, perhaps you can involve them. I've known students who had their partners or special friends help them drill with flash cards (see Survival Skill 7). Others have their children or younger siblings work along with them in drawing and coloring diagrams and sketches. Because you don't want to spend much more than 30 minutes at a time studying anyway (I'll discuss this later), most friends and family members won't object to cooperating with you for a few minutes. In addition, if you're studying with someone you like sharing time with, you're more likely to have fun.

Another way to have fun is to approach your studies with a sense of humor. Draw silly cartoons that illustrate key concepts. Make funny remarks in the margins of your notebook. Set your notes to your favorite melodies. Try thinking of crazy analogies or models for concepts that you're learning. Just have fun with it!

Now let's look at motivation. Sea lions are motivated by fish. Lions are motivated by fresh meat and hugs. My youngest son, Luke, is motivated by hugs, smiles, candy, and Disney World (not in that order). What motivates you? Like most of us, you're probably motivated by a number of different things. How can you tie them into your success in A&P?

More than likely, you're taking this course because it's required for a physical education or health-related career that you're pursuing. Please don't look at this course as simply a hoop you need to jump through (with a C or better) to get a piece of paper that you want. Human A&P is the foundation for *all* of the clinical, therapeutic, and physical professional courses; that is, a *good* understanding of A&P will almost ensure success in your profession. What better motivation is there than this?

Now you may be thinking, "OK, I'm planning a career in physical therapy—why do I need to understand the structure and function of the skin? My motivation for this topic is simply to get the grade." I've been there myself a few times. However, you'd be surprised at how much *everything relates to everything else*. You're right; as a physical therapist you'll probably be focused more on nerves, muscles, and joints than on the skin. However, you'd be surprised how much your understanding of nerves and muscles and joints deepens with an understanding of the concepts behind the structure and function of skin. The trick is that you really can't fully appreciate this link until *you have learned all of it*. In other words, you need to know it before you can begin to understand *why* you need to know it!

Everything relates to everything else.

I hope that you can trust the professionals who designed and required you to take your A&P course and accept the fact that the topics presented in this course really will be important to you—and use that as your motivation to really understand it.

The bottom line to Survival Skill 1 is *know that you can succeed—and you will!*

HINTS

☑ My friend Bill Stark at St. Louis University taught me this trick for making A&P more fun: For each new topic you learn, try to find a song that contains lyrics that relate to the topic—especially if it's a really silly connection or some really outrageous lyrics. Here are some examples:
- Nervous system: *If I Only Had a Brain* (The Wizard of Oz)
- Cardiovascular system: *My Heart Will Go On* (Celine Dion)
- Skeletal system: *Dry Bones* (traditional)
- Urinary system: *Don't Eat the Yellow Snow* (Frank Zappa)
- Reproductive system: *You're Having My Baby* (Paul Anka)

☑ Dr. Stark plays his favorites for the whole class before his lectures. Why not try this yourself? Your professor will probably welcome the contribution; or, perhaps you could have a contest among the people in your study group to come up with the best song.

Know Your Learning Style

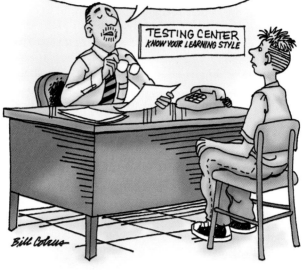

In the previous Survival Skill, we discussed *attitude*. Now let's think about *style*. Learning researchers have found that each of us has a certain style of learning. When we use the word *style* here, it doesn't refer to what kind of clothes we wear to school. Our learning style is the way we approach new information, process that information, and then use it. Familiarity with your own learning style can be a *major* key to success in learning. Knowing your style, you can approach new information in a way that will help you to learn it more efficiently.

Learning styles can be described in many different ways. For example, some learning specialists like to categorize people as being either *left-brain* learners or *right-brain* learners. This system is based on the notion that the part of the brain most involved with complex learning, the cerebrum, is divided into right and left halves. Experiments with patients who have had the connections between these two halves cut by a surgeon show that the right side, acting alone, seems better able to grasp spatial relationships, to interpret nonspeech sounds such as music and animal sounds, and to interpret the sense of touch. The left side seems better able to govern functions of language, such as speaking and writing. Left-brain learners are said to be more logical and mathematical in their approach, whereas right-brain learners tend to be more creative and nonlinear in their approach to learning. Although differences between learners is probably not solely related to the location of brain functions, it's certain that different people learn best in different ways. In addition, using the concepts of left-brain learning and right-brain learning, as well as many other learning concepts, works.

Other approaches to learning style have been proposed—and you should be aware of some of them so that you can better understand the concept of learning style. One approach that I think is very useful is based on how you use your senses in learning. People that learn best by *seeing* a demonstration are called *visual* learners. If you learn better by *hearing* an explanation, then you're probably an *aural* or *auditory* learner. If you need to put your hands on something and *feel* it or work with it, then you're certainly a *kinesthetic* or *tactual* learner. If you learn best by *reading* about something, then you're a *reading* learner. Of course, you might overlap categories. For example, I think that I learn best visually (which explains why I have included so many illustrations in my textbooks and teaching presentations), but I am also strong in the tactual area (which explains why I enjoy teaching in the laboratory).

So why is it important to know your learning style? It's important because if you know your strengths or preferences as a learner, you can arrange your learning activities to build on your strengths. For example, if you're a strong visual learner but are weak in auditory (aural) learning, then you will want to study primarily by drawing diagrams and charting concepts rather than spending most of your time listening to tapes of lectures. On the other hand, a strong auditory (aural) learner will do much better by listening to lecture tapes and spending a little less time with diagrams.

Therefore the first step you must take is to determine *your own style* of learning. You can do this in many ways.

One way to determine your own learning style is to ask a learning specialist to test you. Although formal tests are available, such testing could be as informal as a chat with a staff member at your college's learning center. Another way to discover your own learning style is to ask yourself questions using the self-quiz method.

Here are a few self-quiz questions that will help you to determine your personal approach to learning—that is, your style:

☑ **Do I prefer a verbal explanation of a process or a written explanation?** If you prefer verbal explanations, then concentrate your studies on lectures and verbal dialog with your professor, tutors, members of your study group, and your lab partners. If you prefer written explanations, spend more time with your notes, class handouts, your textbook (yes, please do), and other written materials suggested by your professor or college librarian. You may also want to check out the many resources available on the Internet. (See the special box on computer use in Survival Skill 9.)

☑ **Do I need to see, hear, or touch a model or specimen as I learn about a process?** If you need visuals or something else to hold in your hand, you'll find this course to be just your ticket! A&P involves models, specimens, and other gizmos that you can look at and play with as much as you want. Check with your professor for hints about what kinds of lab models and specimens are available for your studies. In addition, your school library will certainly have many visual and auditory resources, including animations and computer simulations, which might be useful to you.

☑ **Do I learn better at a particular time of the day?** Of course you want to schedule your classes, lab sessions, and study sessions at times when you're at your peak performance level. If you can't do that, then at least take this into consideration and try to break up your study times so that you don't tax your concentration.

☑ **Do I learn better if I am physically active or eating or drinking while I study?** It's always a good idea to take breaks every 15 to 20 minutes while you're studying. When you take a break, move around as much as possible. Considering the benefits of exercise on general physical and mental health (including learning ability and memory), you may want to consider a short walk or a brief stint of lifting weights, doing isometric exercises, or perhaps some floor exercises on your break.

If you like to eat or drink while studying, consider the health consequences. I like to drink while I study, but beer destroys my concentration. Plain old water is absolutely the best thing you can drink while studying! You should be drinking at least eight 8 oz glasses of water a day for good health, anyway. Water prevents dehydration, which can affect your concentration, and it helps your body maintain proper function.

Watch what you eat, too. You don't want to succeed in A&P at the expense of becoming obese! The best snacks are small and frequent, rather than one long eating binge. Depending on your own metabolic system, it's usually best to balance proteins to carbohydrates about 7:9 (protein to carbohydrate), with very little fat. When eating carbohydrates, try to avoid foods very high in complex carbohydrates such as breads, pasta, potato chips, corn chips, and pretzels. Instead use vegetables and fruits that are low in complex carbohydrates. A high ratio of carbohydrates—or too many carbohydrates in a short period of time—will cause your insulin levels to skyrocket and make you feel too sluggish to study effectively.

☑ **Do I prefer starting with the "big picture" and working toward the detail, or do I prefer starting with the detail and assembling the big picture?** At the end of each chapter in nearly every A&P textbook, a section summarizes the important points of the chapter—a sort of *big picture section*. These short, easy-to-read outlines or lists help you put the pieces presented in the text together to see how they fit with one another and allow the body to work as an integrated ("put together") whole. If you like starting with the big picture (which is my style), then move to the back of the chapter and read the last part *first*. Then once you have the big picture in your head, go back to the beginning of the chapter and read the material. If you instead prefer to start with the pieces, then read it just as it's laid out in the book.

These and other questions will help you identify your approach to learning. Once you've done this, you can plan a learning strategy that will process new information in a way that will work best with your learning style. (For free on-line self-quizzes that help you determine your learning style—and advice once you've figured out your style—visit **www.lionden.com/learning_styles.htm**.)

SPECIAL TOPIC: Learners with Special Needs

Unless and until someone with special needs recognizes and names these special needs, learning can be difficult or impossible. I can't think of *any* disability or problem that could prevent someone from learning at least a little about how the body is put together and how it functions.

When dealing with any problem that might affect learning, it's always wise to form a network of support. First, your professor and your college's learning specialists will be able to help you identify your needs if you haven't already pinpointed them; then use these individuals to help you design a strategy to achieve success. I once had a student tell me at the end of two semesters of A&P that she was in fact hearing-impaired, and that she would have probably gotten an *A* instead of a *B* if it were not for

Continued

SPECIAL TOPIC: Learners with Special Needs—cont'd

the fact that I occasionally faced away from her during my lectures and demonstrations (because she was then unable to read my lips). If I had only known at the beginning—if she had *involved me* in her situation—I would have made a conscious effort to make sure that I always faced her and spoke clearly.

It's always wise to form a network of support.

I fully realize that it's often difficult, perhaps even embarrassing, to talk to your professor about your problems—but *that's what we're here for!* Professors have experience, and often some special training, in dealing with a variety of difficulties. When we can't help you, we often know where you can get help; and we are *always* willing to work with you to help you succeed.

Quite a few students have subtle learning problems that they don't recognize—except that they're having some sort of difficulty. I remember one very bright student who really seemed to understand the concepts but just couldn't seem to do better than a *D* on her tests. After helping her all I could with little success, I referred her to our campus learning specialists. Right away they spotted a reading comprehension problem that affected her test-taking ability. Once she developed a new strategy for test-taking, based on her work with a learning specialist, she raised her grade to a final average of *B!* She is now a successful health professional who still uses what she learned that semester to keep up in her field. The important thing is that she took the step of involving others in her situation.

The main thing to remember is that *your special need is part of your learning style.* If you can identify your special needs, you can almost always find a strategy that will help you succeed in learning about human anatomy and physiology (A&P).

HINTS

☑ If you're having *any kind* of difficulty that affects your learning, see your professor or campus learning specialists. Usually these people can help you identify the problem and help you find a strategy to deal with it.

☑ If you already know of a special need that affects your learning, talk to your professor or campus learning specialists *immediately.* The sooner you can form a team to help you with your learning, the better your chances are for great success.

Plan a Learning Strategy

T he intention to learn something is a step in the right direction, but intent alone is not enough for a "learning plan." You must careful-ly plan a set of activities that will move you toward your goals for learning the essentials of human A&P. Consider two important aspects of a good learning strategy: (1) *time management* and (2) *a logical sequence of activities*.

TIME MANAGEMENT

For any plan to work, it must account for timing. A learning strategy must have its foundation in the careful planning of study time for your work in human A&P. To get started, here are a few tips that might help:

☑ **Put your time plan down on paper.** One good way to organize your plan involves three simple steps. First, make a monthly calen-dar. Make or buy a large sheet that shows the whole month at a glance or use one of the many handy monthly planners that you can find at your college bookstore. Those marked "academic" or "fiscal" usually run from July to July and thus work best for the tra-ditional semester or quarter systems. (If your computer or cell phone has a calendar, use that.) Mark your test dates as soon as you know them, as well as days that assignments are due. If your profes-sor has given you dates for particular lecture topics or lab activities, also include them. Be sure to also mark this information for your other classes, as well as other big events and occasions in your life. Do this for the entire semester.

Second, make a weekly schedule. This is an ideal model of a typical week. Include time for your job, your classes, household or personal duties and chores; other commitments such as sports, clubs, or church; time for routine activities such as eating and sleeping; and of course, include plenty of time for studying—mark-ing *specific* times for study each day.

Third, every day make a *to-do* list. This should be a simple list of things you must get done that day. Make your list the evening before or the first thing in the morning. Show which items are high priority and which are low priority and be sure to cross items off your list as you do them. To do this, you need to *carry your list with you all the time.* The easiest way I've found is to use a 3- × 5-inch card. These cards fit almost anywhere and don't tear apart or get lost easily. You can also use your cell phone or personal digital assistant (PDA), if you have one.

☑ **Don't short yourself on study time.** I recommend 1$\frac{1}{2}$ hours *every day* for a typical 3- or 4-credit A&P course. This covers both lecture and lab sections. Some will need more time, and some (especially those using the study skills outlined in later sections) can do with a little less time. If you don't spend enough time working on your studies outside of the classroom, don't expect to be successful—no matter how smart you are. Maybe you didn't need this much time for other courses in high school or college—but A&P is different. You really will need all that time!

If you don't spend enough time working on your studies outside of the classroom, don't expect to be successful—no matter how smart you are.

HINTS

☑ Use the three-step method for time planning:
1. Monthly calendar
2. Weekly schedule
3. Daily *to-do* list

☑ Once you have a plan, FOLLOW IT!

☑ **Break up your study sessions.** Divide your study time into 30-minute blocks if you can. This is the most efficient use of your study time. *Never* go over 90 minutes with study time—the extra time you spend will not do you any good and will probably increase your frustration level. Use unconventional times to do some of your studying. For example, many of my auditory learners listen to taped lectures or study sessions while driving to work or school or doing household chores. I've had several students listen to my taped lectures while working on an assembly line! Others carry their flash cards with them (Survival Skill 7) and review them during unexpected breaks in their day: waiting in lines, just before class starts, and during television commercials.

HINT

☑ Most people can read or concentrate on a topic to be studied for only *20 minutes* at a time! For this reason, frequent breaks and short study sessions always work best.

☑ **Learn when to say "no."** This is the hardest one for me, so I saved it for last. Teachers, like coaches and health professionals, get a kick out of helping people. This is normally a character strength, but if we don't limit ourselves to reasonable schedules, it can become a weakness. While you're studying A&P, you're going to have to put some things off or cancel them entirely—that is, if you want to succeed. Be selective. Say "yes" to important requests and "no" to those that aren't so important. Hanging with your friends is a great thing, and it certainly helps keep stress levels low, but if you say "yes" *too much*, when will you have time to *study*?

Perhaps the most difficult situations occur when your obligations outside of school are simply too demanding to allow your academic success. The wisest decision for some students may be to quit or change a job or temporarily rely on more childcare services than you're usually comfortable with; for others, the best thing to do is to cut back on the course load and lengthen the number of semesters needed to complete the desired program. Often trying to do too much in too little time will guarantee that you will not meet your goals.

LOGICAL SEQUENCE OF ACTIVITIES

The sequence of learning activities within your budgeted study time should be determined by your learning style, any limitations that you may have to live with, and a look at what has worked for others. However, do devise a plan. If you just do study and reading activities in a random manner, you'll be wasting a lot of time. Your overall efficiency is greatly enhanced by using a plan that suits you.

It will take you less time to study if you use an organized plan.

HINTS

☑ If you have trouble budgeting your time, perhaps you should seek the advice of your instructor or a learning specialist.

☑ Ask your librarian about books on time management. Many good titles are available, but you may need your librarian's advice on choosing one that is right for you.

Continued

HINTS—cont'd

☑ Many colleges and local communities offer seminars and workshops on time management. Even those designed primarily for business executives can be extremely helpful to college students.

Here is a plan that has worked for many A&P students:

1. **Read the appropriate chapter in the textbook.** Use a reading strategy that suits your learning style (Survival Skill 5). Don't even try to master it all with this first read-through. Just get a rough idea of what's going on—a fuller understanding will come later. Whatever you do, *don't read more than one chapter at a time!*

2. **Attend the lecture or discussion class, taking careful notes.** Use a note-taking strategy that works for you, as discussed in Survival Skill 6.

3. **Review and organize your notes.** Do this as soon after class as possible—not more than 24 hours. Don't rewrite or copy your notes. That method often does more harm than good.

4. **Participate in related laboratory and demonstration activities.** Try to relate both the lecture and lab sections of the course to the topic—they're complementary courses. If you have the opportunity to do extra lab work or attend extra demonstrations, take advantage of it!

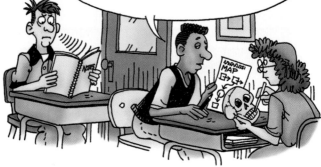

5. **Reread the textbook chapter.** This time through, you'll have a much better understanding of what's going on. Now is the time to highlight, underline, or take notes from the text.

6. **Work through some learning activities.** This is discussed in much greater detail in Survival Skill 7.

7. **Review the material with other students, as in a study group.** This is the most overlooked, but often the *most important*, tip for success in A&P!

8. **Make a quick review of your notes just before the test.** Don't overdo it, though. A lengthy cramming session usually does more harm than good.

SPECIAL TOPIC: Returning Learners

Today more and more people are returning to college and university studies. Traditionally, most college students were recent high school graduates. Returning students who have been out of school for a few (or perhaps many) years are considered "nontraditional" by this standard. Nontraditional students often face challenges that are quite different from those experienced by traditional students.

I've been both a traditional and nontraditional college student myself and have faced many of the challenges you might face while pursuing my college studies: I've worked full-time. I've had the responsibilities of having a spouse and children, and I've also been a single parent. I've worked in a volunteer organization. I've started my own business. I've dealt with divorce, family illnesses, and deaths. I've had personal setbacks and illnesses. I write this to let you know that *I do understand* what some of your challenges are, and I'm here to tell you this: *As overwhelming as it might seem at times, you WILL succeed!*

As overwhelming as it might seem at times—you WILL succeed.

Through the years I've gathered a number of ideas that have helped me or my students face the challenges of being a nontraditional student. Perhaps some of them will be valuable to you.

☑ **Make an informal, *written* contract with your family or life partner.** This simple exercise will help you all understand the seriousness of your commitment to pursue your studies—and each loved one's role in helping you to succeed. It will also avoid the conflict that invariably results from misunderstandings and unspoken expectations.

☑ **Learn to live with dust under the bed, dirty dishes in the sink, and weeds in the garden.** For a time, your priorities will be elsewhere. Don't worry about it. If someone else has a problem with it—well, it's *his* or *her* problem, isn't it?

Continued

SPECIAL TOPIC: Returning Learners—cont'd

☑ **Work with your professor and the learning specialists at your school on strategies for returning learners.** Quite a bit of wisdom is just waiting to be shared with you—but you *have to ask*.

☑ **Find other returning learners with whom you can network.** Many other returning learners would love the mutual support you can provide each other. Sometimes the frustrations can turn to joys when you have a friend with which to share them. If you can include other returning learners in your study group, you might find a special friend there. Often your learning center can refer you to others in your situation. In fact, many schools now have active programs for returning learners. My community college even has a special lounge on campus for returning learners, as well as lunchtime seminars that cover topics of interest to returning learners!

☑ **If possible, postpone big events or life changes until after you're finished with your studies.** If at all possible, don't plan to move, change jobs, change your marital status, have children, undergo a facelift, or try out for the Olympics while you're in school. Life-changing experiences and events can be exciting—but trying to do too many things at the same time while in school can be disastrous!

☑ **Don't hold back.** Some returning learners are somewhat intimidated when they first re-enter the classroom. They don't jump into discussions or speak up with questions. The sooner you realize that the years you've been away from the classroom give you an *advantage* over the younger traditional students, the easier it will be to *jump in* and get the most out of school. A recent study we did at our school showed that out of hundreds of A&P students, those most likely to achieve a high grade were the older students!

Arrange a Suitable Study Area

J ust as the timing of study activities is important, the location in which you work can be critical to your success in learning A&P effectively. Because none of us lives in an ideal world, you may have to settle for less than the best. However, extra effort put into securing a prime study site could pay big dividends at test time.

The following things should be considered when selecting a study location:

☑ **Make sure you have good access to the site.** Don't plan to study in an area that is closed during your planned study time or that is often being used by others before you get there. In addition, if you're hosting a study group, make sure that you choose a convenient location. If you live way out in the boonies and all your study partners live in town, then find somewhere midway to meet them.

☑ **Be sure that you have comfortable lighting.** Some learners do best in bright lighting, others in moderately dim lighting. Despite all the stories you've heard about Abe Lincoln studying by the light of the fireplace in his cabin, very dim light is not good for studying. Likewise, you may find reading easier in incandescent rather than fluorescent lighting—especially if you have a reading disability. If you have any difficulty with your vision while studying, or experience headaches as a result, talk to your physician or eye-care professional.

☑ **Ensure that the surroundings complement your learning style.** In other words, make sure that your site is comfortable. However, make sure it's not so comfortable that you'll tend to doze!

☑ **Analyze the background noise.** Few study locations are perfectly noiseless. Ask yourself whether your selected site has noise that will be tolerable (loud or soft; people sound, music sound, or machine sound).

☑ **Make sure you have what you need to study.** If you need pens, pencils, paper, computer, disks, video player, live band, books, tapes, basketball, or whatever, make sure you have them *before you begin to study.*

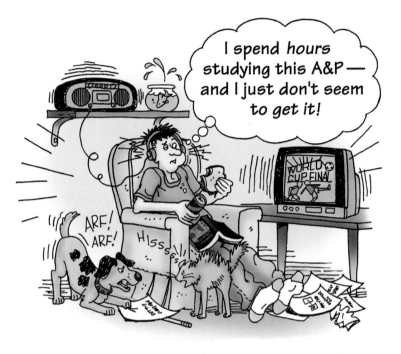

HINT

☑ Can't think of a good place to study? Try the following 12 places:

1. College library
2. Public library
3. Student lounge
4. Campus quad
5. Local park
6. Campus study room
7. Bedroom
8. Café
9. Work (if your boss permits it)
10. Parent room at a play spot
11. Yard near your home
12. Front porch

Plan a Reading Strategy

Although reading the right chapter is one element of the overall learning strategy, reading requires a strategy of its own. In the case of A&P textbooks, especially, the "jump right into it" approach used for novels or magazine articles does not work very well. Instead you must do some *prereading* and *postreading* of a new chapter if you're to understand it well.

Learning specialists have invented several reading strategies. A popular method that works well with most A&P textbooks is called the *SQ4R Reading Method.* The six steps of this method (Survey, Question, Read, Recite, Record, Review) are described below:

1. **SURVEY the chapter before you read it.** That is, glance over the start-of-chapter materials (such as word lists or brief outlines); then glance over the body of the chapter (paying more attention to the topic headlines, tables, and illustrations than the actual narrative), and the end-of-chapter materials (summary information). Leave the end-of-chapter questions or problems for a later step.

HINT

☑ You may have heard about famous successful people, such as U.S. presidents, taking special training in reading to improve their speed and comprehension. Check out the many reading programs that are probably available in your area. If it worked for John F. Kennedy, it ought to work for you, too!

2. **Ask yourself QUESTIONS.** Ask WHAT, WHY, and HOW as you survey the chapter, as you read the chapter, and after you're finished reading. Asking such questions will help you find answers as you read—thereby helping you focus on the important ideas.

Always be willing to challenge what the textbook author(s) present to you in the text (just don't challenge us to a duel!). Doing this will help you develop critical thinking skills. Take your challenges to your study group or professor—it may spark a discussion that will really help you understand more deeply.

3. **READ the chapter.** As you read, look for the main ideas and how they're organized. Textbook authors put a lot of thought into how our chapters are organized, always building in a progression that we think will help you see the big picture. Try to get a feel for the rhythm and pace of the writing style. In addition, don't forget the tables, illustrations, and boxed sections. Much to our editors' dismay, textbook authors often leave certain things out of the narrative but instead put them into tables or illustrations where we think they make more sense. You'll miss these important ideas if you read only the narrative. (Remember, don't expect to "get it" all on your first read through. This is very technical stuff; it takes a few tries to really get it.)

HINTS

- ☑ Concentrate on what you're reading. If you can't concentrate, then put the book down and come back to it later. Don't waste your time!
- ☑ Don't highlight or mark the text yet! That comes later.
- ☑ Some readers do well in understanding the connection between text and illustration by using the two-finger approach: using one finger to follow the text and the other to trace elements of the figure.

Unlike a novel, which you just read through, a textbook should be bitten off in pieces. Don't move to the next section until you've taken the time to stop and consider each **boldface term.** Textbook authors take the trouble to highlight them because THEY'RE IMPORTANT! In addition, take the time to make sure you answer any end-of-section review items before moving to the next section.

4. **RECITE aloud what you have just read.** When my daughter Aileen was first learning to read, she used to often recap aloud what she had just finished reading. No wonder her comprehension was so remarkable (do I sound like a proud Dad, or what?). When I first tried this method, I felt pretty silly—like a little kid. However, you don't have to speak loudly, and it *really does help*. Recap aloud what you've read after each page or section—don't wait until the end of the chapter or this tip won't help you.

5. **RECORD the main ideas.** Some people prefer to use a highlighting pen to highlight important terms and phrases as a method of

recording the main ideas for future use. You can go back later and review the portions you've highlighted. If you choose the highlighting method, make sure you don't highlight everything—or it won't be very useful to you. You might also try writing yourself notes in the margins. I don't like this method much myself; I find it more effective to write down the main ideas in a special "reading notebook" that I keep. If you're an auditory (aural) learner, you might want to record your thoughts verbally into a small tape recorder for later review. Whatever you do, *use your own words* as you write, don't simply parrot the text.

6. **REVIEW your textbook and reading notes often.** Review what you've read *every day*. As you review your own notes, compare them against the summary material at the end of the chapter. If you do this, an understanding of the material will seem to come to you rather effortlessly. When you review, don't try to focus on a complete understanding at first—it will progress with continued reviewing. If you're not progressing, see your professor for help in getting on the right track.

After you've reviewed the chapter and your notes a few times, you're ready to tackle the end-of-chapter material in earnest. It's best to write out the answers to the questions or problems—or recite them aloud. If you just "think them through" without *actively* responding, you won't learn as quickly or efficiently.

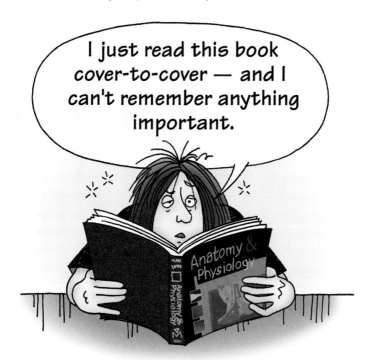

HINTS

☑ If you choose the highlighting method of recording, try using different colors of highlighting pens for different topics or different kinds of information or different levels of importance.

☑ Some learners use Post-It® notes in margins or as page tabs as they record. These come in different styles and colors. Play around with them and see if you can develop your own customized system!

☑ Many similar methods of textbook reading exist, one of which might serve you better. Here are two:
  1. PQRST (Preview, Question, Read, Summarize, Test)
  2. OK5R (Overview, Key ideas, Read, Record, Recite, Review, Reflect)

☑ You can find details about these and other reading strategies at your college learning center or library, or visit www.lionden.com/reading. htm.

6

Analyze Your Note-Taking Skills

A s you may know, taking notes during a lecture or discussion improves both comprehension (understanding) and retention (recall) of information. Because note taking requires on-the-spot organization of data seen and heard during the class period, it improves *comprehension*. Because note taking reinforces information as it's recorded, it improves *retention*. Here are a few points to consider when planning a note-taking strategy:

Note taking is the key to comprehension, retention, and recall.

☑ **Know the professor's style.** Some professors present A&P in a well-organized manner, whereas others tend to ramble. Some speak very softly—or perhaps too loudly. Some may choose to follow the organization of the textbook very closely; others may decide to take a completely different approach. Being conscious of a professor's style will help you determine how you want to organize your notes, whether you'll need a tape recorder to back up your notes, and where you want to sit in the classroom.

HINTS

☑ If your professor rambles during lectures, leave wide spaces between entries in your notebook. That way, if the professor returns to a previous point, you have room to fill in more points.

☑ If your professor follows the textbook closely (bless his or her heart!), have the textbook handy and highlight key points in it as you take notes. However, don't substitute highlighting for writing notes—you'll be sorry if you do!

☑ **Plan for note taking.** Know what style of note taking you will rely on, what materials you need to have with you, and how much lap or desktop space you require. Make sure that you're ready to start writing *before the professor begins class.*

☑ **Listen well.** Before you can take effective notes, you must **hear** what is being presented. This means making sure not only that you can perceive the sound but also that you understand the meaning. Try to clue in on the speaker's personal style to determine the main points and relationships between concepts.

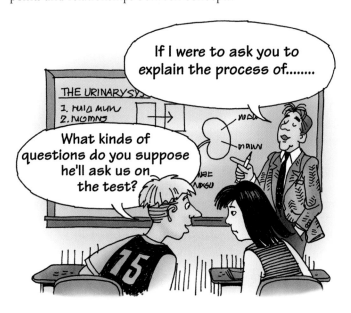

Most professors give a lot of clues that will help you. For example, if the professor says, "If I asked you to describe the function of a lysosome, what would you tell me?" then I bet he is thinking of asking something like that on a test or quiz. At the very least, the professor has raised an important question for you to think about. It amazes me how often in class I come right out and say, "I often ask this on a test," and watch as most of my students make no notation of this in their notebooks! It's no surprise that those who do take note of these comments always get those particular test items correct.

☑ **Structure your notes.** Because note taking helps you organize the contents of a lecture, make sure that you're conscious of structure as you proceed.

   1. *Know ahead of time whether you will use a formal outline style or your own personal modified outline style.* Here are some possible styles for note taking. You can use any of the outline formats

shown here—or invent one that suits you! Be creative and invent your own personal style of outlining!

Formal outline:

I. Heading
   A. Subtopic
   B. Subtopic
      1. More about the subtopic
      2. More about the subtopic
         a. Greater detail
         b. Greater detail
            (1) Even more detail
            (2) Even more detail

Modified formal outline:

1. Heading
   a. Subtopic
   b. Subtopic
      i. More about the subtopic
      ii. More about the subtopic
         (1) Greater detail
         (2) Greater detail
            (a) Even more detail
            (b) Even more detail

Legal-style outline:

I. Heading
   I.1 Subtopic
   I.2 Subtopic
      1.2.1 More about the subtopic
      1.2.2 More about the subtopic
         1.2.2.1 Greater detail
         1.2.2.2 Greater detail
            1.2.2.2.1 Even more detail
            1.2.2.2.2 Even more detail

Bulleted outline:

• Heading
   ○ Subtopic
   ○ Subtopic
      ➤ More about the subtopic
      ➤ More about the subtopic
         ■ Greater detail
         ■ Greater detail
            ✳ Even more detail
            ✳ Even more detail

2. *Be concise.* Don't try to take down every word, but use phrases, abbreviations, symbols, and diagrams to summarize the points made by the lecturer. For example, use *Ca* or *Ca*$^{++}$ for calcium, *w/*for with, *w/o* for without, # for number, ★ for something that is likely to be a test item, and *Enz* for enzyme—just to name a few. However, make sure you know what your symbol or short-hand means later on, when it's not so fresh in your memory!

3. *Leave room between entries.* This way you can fill in more infor-mation if the professor returns to a point. Another method is to use only the right or left half of your notepaper. Some students fold each page of notes in half lengthwise to form a margin down the middle. That leaves a lot of room for adding things later.

4. *Try using highlighting pens or colored pencils to organize notes with color.* Use Post-It® notes or tabs in a similar way (a variety of colors, shapes, and sizes exist).

☑ **Process your notes.** As soon after a lecture as possible (within 24 hours), work with your notes to clarify what you wrote. Fill in blank spots you may have left, and write out abbreviated terms so that you'll know the meaning later. Don't completely rewrite or transcribe your notes, but be sure that everything is there and is understandable. If you find a gap or muddled section, check with a classmate or the lecturer for clarification.

Don't completely rewrite or transcribe your notes.

☑ **Write it out!** The most common error in note taking is being too brief. Write out complete thoughts, not just key words or phrases. Draw diagrams or sketches if that helps you understand the materi-al. Write *as much as you can* during the class, and you'll thank yourself later. If you can't keep up with a fast-talking professor, then (with permission) tape the presentation and go over your notes later with other students. In addition, write legibly—you want to be able to read it later!

☑ **Look for connections.** One of the great secrets in really under-standing A&P is looking for how things are related to one anoth-er—connections. Your note-taking system can be used to recognize and keep track of connections in a number of ways.

The easiest way is to keep a section of your notebook, perhaps tabbed so you can find it easily, for "connection pages." On the top of each connection page, write the name of a concept that keeps coming up in the course; then as you process your regular notes, when you run across that concept again, add the new information to your connection page for that topic. For example, calcium has a variety of important roles in the body and will be discussed frequently. Every time calcium comes up in the discussion, add it to your "calcium page" in the "connections section" of your notebook. You'll probably end up with a lock-and-key page, sodium page, G-protein page, sodium-cotransport page, citric acid cycle page, cytoskeleton page, collagen page, and receptor page. (For more ideas about connection pages, visit **www.lionden.com/ concept_lists.htm**.)

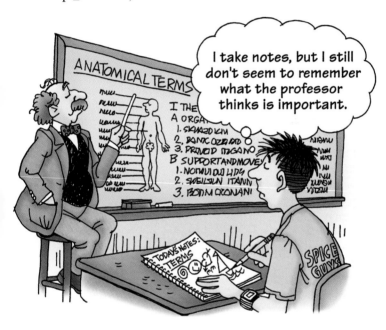

Study Actively

Many students feel that studying is the same as reading, so they spend study time only in reading and rereading the textbook and class notes. Although reading is a part of a study plan, additional activities are required for your study time to be *effective*. Here are a few aggressive supplements to add to your study regimen:

☑ **Answer the review questions found at the end of each chapter.** Write out the answers; don't just answer them in your head.

☑ **Do some or all of the activities in the study guide.** Often a study guide will accompany your A&P textbook that will provide you with specific activities to work through the concepts of each chapter.

HINT

☑ The language of A&P really is a foreign language! It's mostly Latin. Although some word parts also come from Greek, German, and other languages, almost all the terms are in Latinized form. It really helps with vocabulary if you take a look at the word parts and their meanings, too. Many of my students have added this feature to their flash cards—and swear by it. To find the word parts for any term, refer to *Mosby's Medical, Nursing, and Allied Health Dictionary* (which is available in both print and compact disc [CD] versions) or refer to the list of word parts in your A&P textbook.

☑ **Keep up with the new vocabulary.** A number of years ago, a language professor published an article that stated that A&P students learn more new words than students in a freshman foreign language course! By far, the easiest way to work on vocabulary is by making and using flash cards. Write the term on one side of an index card and the meaning on the reverse side. Then simply review the deck of cards you'll have for each chapter. Don't try to cram with these cards, just look at the word, try to remember the meaning, then check yourself by flipping the card over. Carry the deck with you and review them when you have a minute now and then. Some students tape their flash cards all over their homes so that they're constantly reviewing the material. If you tackle them gradually but frequently, you'll know all the important terms with hardly any effort!

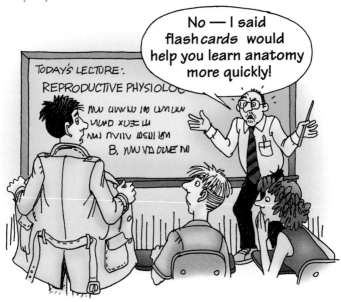

Test your creativity by devising other vocabulary-strengthening activities. However, don't make the mistake of thinking that if you've mastered the vocabulary, you have a complete understanding of the topic. Vocabulary building is the *foundation*, not the whole thing. For more help in learning new terminology, visit **www.lionden.com/new_terms.htm**.

☑ **Use computer-assisted tutorials, visualizations, or reviews.** Some textbooks come with a CD or link to a set of on-line study resources. Some of these are sort of like computer games—making studying a little more fun. In addition, many stand-alone programs can be purchased or may be available in your college learning center or library. (Check the special box on using the computer to study A&P in this guide for more hints.)

☑ **Form a study group.** Get together with others in your course to discuss, review, and process A&P together. Ask each other test questions that you devise yourselves; argue about the correct answers. Meet on a regular basis throughout the semester, not just before big tests or exams. Believe it or not, research shows that study groups are one of the most effective learning strategies we know! It helps if you have a group with mixed levels of natural talent or previous experience with the subject. The better students will learn more by teaching the weaker students; the weaker students will benefit from the peer tutoring by the better students. However, any mix of students should work.

Study groups are one of the most effective learning strategies.

How do you find study partners? I guess taking out an ad in the *Personals* section of the college paper might work, but the best way is to just ask your lab partners or the people sitting near you in your A&P class if they would like to join a study group with you. If they're already in one, ask if you can join. If you're having trouble finding study partners, ask your professor or learning center to help. In addition, please listen to the voice of experience: Asking someone to be your study partner when your real goal is dating is *not a good idea!* (For more advice on group study, please visit **www.lion-den.com/ study_groups.htm**.)

☑ **Make a "concept map" of important concepts.** A *concept map* is a graphic representation of an idea that can take many forms. Here are a few examples of the different kinds of concept maps you might try:

1. *Flow chart.* A flow chart, such as the one shown on page 59 (Figure 1-4) of this book, shows the step-by-step process of building a protein. Figure 4-15 on page 245 shows yet another, simpler, style that pulls together many different concepts into one chart about blood flow. Many other examples of flow diagrams are provided in this book and in your textbook. How many can you find?

2. *Circle diagram.* A circle diagram is really just a flow chart in a circular arrangement. This is a favorite style among biologists, because so many biologic processes are cycles (circles). Look at the examples on page 91 (Figure 1-12) in this book. Notice how the circle diagram is like a snake biting its tail: you always return to where you started.

3. *Tree diagram.* A tree diagram is really just an outline of topics and subtopics. To produce an outline such as the outline or summary found at the end of each textbook chapter, you have to know the organization and relationship of all the ideas involved

in a topic—a great way to improve your understanding. If you incorporate sketches in your outline, you'll be even closer to a full understanding.

4. *Full-color sketch.* A sketch of a concept, especially if it involves colors, really kicks a lot of senses into gear to help you learn a concept. I know one student who draws out some concepts as a series of cartoon panels, as you might see in a comic book. I'm still pitching my editors with the idea that I'll someday produce a comic book version of our A&P text! Hey, if it works for *Classics Illustrated* and *Scientific American*—why not?

5. *Tables.* Create tables such as those found in Part 2 of this book. Such tables help you draw information together in ways that shows you *connections* between ideas.

Be creative! Build concept maps out of clay, dough, or craft sticks. Paint a watercolor of the cell. Photograph or videotape your study partners acting out the citric acid cycle. Use your computer to animate the function of muscle cells. Have fun with it!

Your professor, learning center, or library will be able to help you learn how to do concept mapping, or you can visit **www.lion den.com/concept_maps.htm**.

HINTS

☑ Dr. Tom Westfall, my department chair at St. Louis University Medical School and a popular, award-winning teacher of pharmacology, suggests that his students learn drug names, their pharmacologic classifications, and their actions by incorporating them into lyrics that can be sung to well-known melodies.

☑ When you have a particularly difficult concept or list of facts to deal with, try composing a poem or song that will help you learn it. The act of composing will help you organize your thoughts and understanding of the subject, and repeating the poem or song can help you remember the essential elements of the concept.

☑ Drawing diagrams and pictures of concepts is a great way to increase your understanding of those concepts. I've found that to be true as I sketch out the art concepts that I give to the illustrators of the textbook. My understanding is always clearer after drawing a picture or diagram because *I have to get the relationships right* before I can finish the picture.

☑ If you come up with a new idea for a diagram, table, or illustration tÀ@really helps you, send it to me. I may use your idea in the next edition of this book!

Use All Your Resources

S
ome learning resources are obvious: the textbook, the study guide, your notes, the professor, the course syllabus, and so on. Other useful resources are often less obvious, so allow me to list some (so you don't miss any):

☑ Teaching assistants, aides, and tutors (some colleges and universities provide tutors free of charge)

☑ Study partners (classmates)

☑ Friends who have recently taken the A&P course

☑ Campus learning center or library

☑ Other A&P books (references, texts)

☑ Related journal, newspaper, or magazine articles (*Science News*, *Discover*, and *Scientific American* are particularly useful for A&P students—but now would also be a good time to start reading professional journal articles to prepare you for your professional career.)

☑ Television (Series such as Nova and Scientific American, as well as news magazines and special series on Public Broadcasting System [PBS], The Learning Channel [TLC], and Discovery Channel, are great resources. Check your college library or bookstore for videos that might help you.)

☑ Study skills courses, seminars, and books on study skills

HINTS

☑ If you ever see the film *Fantastic Voyage* in your television listings or on a shelf at the video store, watch it! The special effects are really cheesy by today's standards, even though they won the film an Academy Award in 1966. However, the effects are good enough to show a neat concept for visualizing the inside of the human body. Use this imagery yourself and take an imaginary fantastic voyage as you learn microscopic A&P.

HINTS—cont'd

☑ EPCOT Center at Disney World in Orlando, Florida, has a great ride based on this film. It's called *Body Wars*. If you're at Disney World, tear yourself away from Mickey long enough to go on this ride!

SPECIAL TOPIC: Using Your Computer to Study A&P

More and more students have access to computers today. Personal computers, school and library computers, and computers at your workplace have made these tools widely available. We haven't really had time to develop a cultural mindset on using computers regularly to learn, but that is rapidly changing! I've listed just a few of the many ways to use a computer here. Perhaps they'll give you some new ideas for using this tool to learn A&P.

☑ **Keep your notes on a word processor.** Don't rewrite your class notes, but keep a separate set of notes that combines information from your class notes, lab notes, text reading notes, and study session notes. Some students bring notebook or palmtop computers to class to take notes. I don't think this is a good idea *unless you're very fast with your computer*. In any case, always have a paper notebook handy to draw diagrams and sketches!

☑ **Use a flow-charting program to make concept maps.** Some of these programs are intended for business organizations and computer programmers but can be used for concept maps. You can also use illustration, drawing, and presentation programs for concept mapping. Simple painting or drawing programs that are probably on your computer somewhere can also be very useful for making concept maps.

☑ **Use programs specifically designed for learning A&P.** You may have a CD enclosed with your textbook, which is a great way to explore some of the topics in A&P. Many publishers publish stand-alone A&P software. Research your choice carefully. Not all programs are as useful as they first appear! For example, some are geared for advanced students and some for professionals.

☑ **Use programs that are not specifically for A&P.** Elsevier and other publishers have a variety of computer programs in related topics that may help you with A&P. For example, medical terminology and medical dictionary programs or databases will help you learn the language of A&P. Medical, nursing, or allied health titles might help, as will certain health, physical education, and sports titles. General study skills programs might be useful, too.

Continued

SPECIAL TOPIC: **Using Your Computer to Study A&P—cont'd**

☑ **Use the Internet.** A variety of resources are available on the Internet today. You can use search engines such as Google, Yahoo!, or Answers.com to search for topics that you're studying. However, be careful—many resources exist, and finding a useful one may take a long time. Often your textbook's website, or your course's website, will have links or other resources that are more likely to help you. (For a starting place that links to a variety of different A&P websites, try my website at lionden. com/ap.htm.)

☑ **Use e-mail, instant messaging, and chat rooms.** Personal communication on the Internet really makes studying in a group practical— even when you can't meet face to face. In addition, it's a great way to communicate with your professor!

☑ **Use your course web resources.** Increasingly, course management tools like WebCT, Blackboard, and others are being used in A&P courses. These platforms frequently have links constructed by your professor, discussion forums, chat rooms, class e-mail lists, and more.

Prepare for Tests

Obviously, you prepare for tests by studying the appropriate course material. However, a few special tricks may help you deal with the testing situation itself. Here are some of the tips I have found useful:

☑ **Practice taking the test.** Sometimes professors provide sample questions or old editions of an A&P test. Sample test questions may also appear in the study guide available to accompany your textbook. If you anticipate test questions in the style that your professor uses, which you can do after a test or two, you can then make up your own questions and use them on each other in your study group.

HINTS

☑ Practice taking essay tests by anticipating questions (such as those at the back of each chapter in the textbook) and *writing out the answers*.

☑ My friend and former composition teacher Ron Giedinghagen always made us write all of our practice essays in a 50-minute class. This forced us to learn how to sketch out our ideas, organize our points, write the darn thing, and proofread in the shortest possible time. Practice writing essays under timed conditions and you'll gain a very valuable skill—and you'll find yourself thinking more clearly when facing test questions.

☑ **Stay healthy.** Don't overtax yourself in studying (especially last-minute cramming) to a point that makes you sick, sleepy, or otherwise unable to operate at peak efficiency. Many students use extra caffeine or other stimulants to keep them awake as they study the

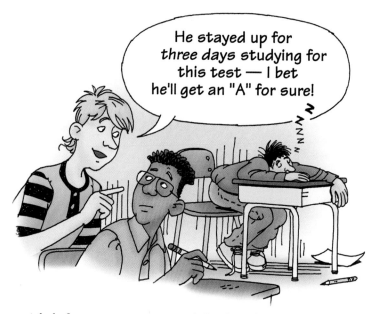

night before an exam — or even while taking the test. If you take caffeine (in coffee or soft drinks, for example) then use the normal amount and stay away from other stimulants.

☑ **Be comfortable.** Within the limits of your particular situation, dress as comfortably as possible and find a portion of the test room that suits you. Don't wear new shoes or a pair of slacks that is too tight on test day!

☑ **Anticipate stress.** No matter how confident you may feel, the test situation is stressful. The stress that you experience may negatively influence your performance on a particular test. Knowing that ahead of time, you can form a plan for what to do if you feel pressured during the exam. Closing your eyes and calmly counting 10 slow breaths may help, as might concentrating on a relaxing image. You may even consider participating in one of the test anxiety workshops held on many campuses.

HINT

☑ Prepare mnemonic devices (memory helpers) to help you learn lists of concepts. I have more on this method later, in the boxed section on student laboratories.

☑ **Make a final review of important concepts.** This review should be just a refresher right before the test. It should not be the first time you look at the material in preparation for the test. Cramming is very seldom an effective strategy.

Cramming is not an effective strategy.

Use a Test-Taking Strategy During the Examination

O nce you have begun the examination, you should still be implementing a strategy. Test-taking is more than just passively spewing forth information. It's a process that requires thought, skill, and action. A&P students have found these hints useful:

☑ **Read the instructions.** Really. So many students don't read the directions to a test because they're so anxious to get moving on the test itself. However, often the instructions include key items that will help you take it—and avoid frustrations of not being able to figure out how to fill out your test forms.

☑ **Know the testing style.** Do what you can to find out specifics of the test's construction (format of the test, number of items, time given to complete the test, wording of the test items, and level of complexity).

☑ **Skim over the test before answering any questions.** Remember, read the directions for the entire test first. Then briefly look at the style and content of all the questions. It only takes a couple of minutes, and you'll know exactly what you're up against.

☑ **Skip questions that stump you.** If you come across a puzzling question, save it for later (when you know better how much time you can devote to it). It's not worth fretting over one question when it's eating up time you could be spending on questions that you're able to answer well.

☑ **Know how to evaluate objective items logically.** Your college learning center should be able to provide some help in learning how to apply principles of logic to objective tests. If you can't find help there, ask your librarian. Librarians *always* know where to find help!

☑ **Understand the nature of each item.** Is it fill-in, matching, or multiple-choice? Are there any special instructions? Is there more than one correct answer; can the same answer appear more than once? Must the answer be in complete sentences?

☑ **Analyze the wording.** Watch for key qualifying words such as *all, every, always, never, sometimes, often, usually.* Underline them. Absolute qualifiers such as *always* and *never* in a TRUE/FALSE item usually make the statement false. Determine whether the answer should be singular or plural, as well as the part of speech (noun, verb, adverb, adjective). If any part of a TRUE/FALSE item is false, *then the entire statement is false.* In essay questions or short-answer questions, look for key words such as *compare* (tell how things are alike), *contrast* (tell how things are different), *interpret* (give your explanation or meaning), and *discuss* (give a complete account). Your campus learning center may have a list of such words, as well as their exact meanings.

☑ **Eliminate choices.** If several choices are offered (or occur to you) and all seem likely to be correct, try to eliminate those that are *least likely.* Such analysis may trigger a thought that leads you to the correct choice.

☑ **If you have to, guess.** If blank answers are scored the same as wrong guesses and you're really stumped, guess anyway, because (assuming you studied) your answer will be an *informed* guess, which is certainly better than a blank.

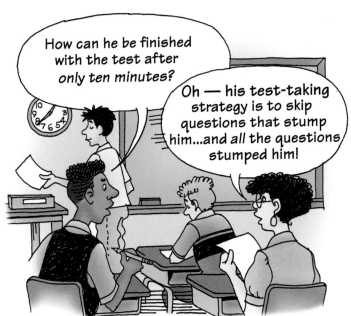

How can he be finished with the test after only ten minutes?

Oh — his test-taking strategy is to skip questions that stump him...and all the questions stumped him!

☑ **Plan your answers.** Essay and short-answer questions require a logical presentation if you want the maximum points from the grader. I find it easiest to jot down a brief outline of the answer first—just phrases that summarize the main points. Take a quick look at your micro-outline. Do the points flow in a logical order, leading to your main point? If not, rearrange them. Once you have a clear micro-outline, write out your answer.

☑ **Understand the directions.** This is especially important for this type of item, because it will determine the approach you take in planning a response. Amazingly, many students *don't even read the directions!* How much more strongly can I emphasize this? Don't assume you know how the professor wants you to fill out the test just because you recognize the format. There's the famous story of the incredibly difficult exam that one student finished, with a perfect score, in only 2 minutes. The directions on that test ended with the phrase, "and only answer one item, of your choosing, out of the 200 items given here." Only that one student bothered to read the directions thoroughly enough to see it. I think this is probably one of those mythical campus legends, but it makes a good point!

☑ **Understand the question.** Although key words are important, they're not the question itself. Take some time to mull over the question to be sure that you know what the question asks. If you don't understand the question, or if you don't understand the directions, then ask your professor or the test proctor. Unless you've been instructed not to ask questions, any question you ask is worth asking—it might make the difference in whether you answer correctly.

☑ **Start with a thesis statement.** A thesis statement is simply a sentence that summarizes the core of your answer succinctly. Usually a rephrasing of the question makes a suitable thesis statement.

☑ **Arrange your points logically.** After stating your thesis, support it by a series of paragraphs (or sentences) that back it up. Organize them in a manner that presents the material in the most convincing way possible.

☑ **If possible, make a concluding statement.** A restatement of the thesis (although not in exactly the same words) works best. A concluding remark is good style, and it allows you to emphasize your main point.

☑ **Don't dance around the central issue.** Many students feel that weaving circles around an issue that they don't understand completely will fool the grader into believing that they do understand it. It's likely that the grader will not only see that critical content is missing but also will become irritated with the student. Irritating the grader is not a good strategy for subjectively graded items!

HINT

☑ My friend Mary Ellen McDonald gives her students this nifty
R-A-C-E-S method for dealing with multiple-choice items:
<u>R</u>ead the question carefully.
<u>A</u>nalyze the question to see what's really being asked.
<u>C</u>ircle any words that might affect the meaning of the question
(such as *except*, *not*).
<u>E</u>liminate as many choices as you can.
<u>S</u>elect the best choice from the remaining items.

HINTS

☑ For more help on test-taking strategies and resources, visit www.
lionden.com/test-taking.htm.
☑ For strategies in taking on-line tests, visit www.lionden.com/
online_tests.htm.

SPECIAL TOPIC: The Student Laboratory

The laboratory portion of the typical A&P course is in some ways
a unique beast. I've collected a few ideas on how to make the student laboratory the best possible experience:

☑ **Safety is always first!** Do you remember me mentioning that I used
to be a lion tamer? Lion tamers are sticklers for safety. Lion taming
seems like a foolhardy and reckless occupation, but the reality is far
different. Lion tamers never take a step into the cage without every
possible safety precaution being in place. Absolute tyrants about safety! Why? Because one little mistake often means death. My friends the
Flying Wallendas of high-wire fame are the same way about safety precautions. The only people that I know of that are pickier about safety
are scientists (for the same reason). A mistake in the lab, even a student lab, can make you as dead as my friend, Wayne Franzen, who was
killed by one of his tigers a few years ago, or Karl Wallenda, when he
fell to his death from the high wire back when I was an undergradu-
ate. I've seen far too many preventable injuries in student labs—
they're awful. So PLEASE heed all the safety precautions printed in
your lab manuals, posted in your labs, and articulated or published by
your school or professor or both. In addition, use common sense.

Continued

SPECIAL TOPIC: The Student Laboratory—cont'd

☑ **Use the "field method" for identifying anatomic structures.** Roger Tory Peterson, the famous naturalist and birder, developed a method for field identification of birds that has since been used for everything from identifying sparrows to spotting enemy aircraft. The Peterson method focuses on "field marks," the one or two characteristics that distinguish particular birds or airplanes from similar birds or airplanes. I used this method to tell the difference between my lions: one had a scar on the nose, another a notch in the ear, yet another an odd color to his mane. Simply approach tissues, bones, bone markings, muscles, and other structures that you need to identify in lab courses as you would animals in the field. Focus on the one or two characteristics that make one tissue different from all others. Peterson's method also makes use of range maps that show where different birds are likely to be found. Do the same with lab specimens. Where are adductor muscles likely to be found? On the inside of limbs. So where would you start looking for *adductor longus?* Use a little tip from field geography, too. It might take you all day to find the Mississippi River on a map if you have no clue what a river is. When learning bone markings, how can you find the supraorbital foramen when you have no idea what a foramen is? Study types of things, like types of muscles, types of bones, and so on, before studying the specific examples assigned to you.

☑ **Remember that the laboratory is a playground.** That doesn't mean you should just goof around for no good reason. It does mean that labs are intended to be fun, hands-on opportunities to play with specimens, models, and experimental equipment. Therefore, approach it that way. Don't just try to get by with the minimum activity. If you linger and look a little deeper, or turn the model around this way, then another way, you'll find a deeper understanding of what you were supposed to find, as well as the connections that help you draw concepts together into the *big picture.* Kinesthetic (tactual) learners will especially benefit from this aspect of the lab course—often in ways that bring home points from the lecture or discussion portions of the course.

☑ **Use flash cards.** Flash cards are especially useful in certain lab activities. My students like to draw pictures of lab specimens on one side of a card and its name or description on the other side. I even had one student who brought in a camera and took photos of her dissections so that she could make flash cards! Your cell phone may have a camera—use it as a learning tool in lab!

☑ **Use mnemonic devices.** Archeologists have recently uncovered evidence that mnemonic devices were used by the ancient Greeks thousands of years ago in their famous schools. You may have seen one of

SPECIAL TOPIC: The Student Laboratory—cont'd

those famous memory experts that can spout off all the names on a page in the phone book using mnemonic devices. Mnemonic devices are little sayings or mental images you use to help you remember a concept. For example, the acronym *IPMAT* has been used by generations of students to help them learn the phases of the cell cycle: interphase, prophase, metaphase, anaphase, and telophase. The mnemonic sentence "On old Olympus's tiny tops, a friendly Viking grew vines and hops," is listed in this book as a mnemonic for learning the names (in order) of the 12 pairs of cranial nerves. Each word in the phrase begins with the same letter as the name of a cranial nerve. You can find it in the note following Table 3-8. A far raunchier version exists that I won't share here, but maybe you can figure one out. The sillier the phrase or mental image you use, or the more ribald, the easier it is to remember and the more useful it is as a memory aid.

☑ **Dissect like an artist.** Some of the best anatomists have in fact also been great artists. I don't know of any anatomists that were also axe murderers. I don't think this is purely coincidental. Artistic finesse in pulling apart structures without destroying them or removing them from their relative position in the body is far more effective than the hacking style of an axe murderer. Your goal is to find structures so that you can understand how the body is constructed, not to make hamburger in the shortest possible time.

Continued

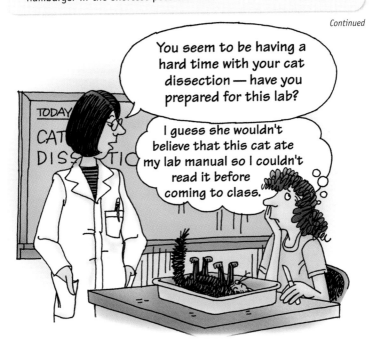

SPECIAL TOPIC: The Student Laboratory—cont'd

☑ **You don't have to be a great sketch artist.** However, you should *sketch a lot*. Draw everything! Don't sweat and slave over creating a masterpiece—even if you're capable of creating a masterpiece (wait until after lab and work on your masterpiece on the weekend). However, do take enough time with it that you can recognize key features later on when you use your sketches to study. In addition, label as much as you can. A sketch without any labels is pretty useless; except maybe as a coaster.

☑ **Come to the lab prepared.** Read what you will be doing in lab *before you do it*. If you don't come prepared, then half the time spent in the lab will be spent just trying to figure out what to do. The other half of your time will be spent trying to rush through the activity without any appreciation of the concepts behind it. Preparation also means reading the portions of the textbook that relate to the lab activity. Preparation is probably the greatest key to using the student lab to its greatest potential.

☑ **Use many resources.** When you're trying to find anatomic specimens or interpret results from a physiology demonstration or experiment, don't rely solely on your textbook and lab manual. Often your specimen will not look like the picture in these books. No organ or tissue looks exactly like any other. Therefore find out where you can purchase or borrow a lab atlas, anatomy atlas, histology book, and other useful resources. In addition, many useful resources for A&P lab can be found on the Internet (you can use a search engine to find them).

HINT

☑ My friend Mary Ellen McDonald offers the F-I-R-S-T strategy for developing mnemonic sentences:

F̲orm a word.

I̲nsert the letters.

R̲earrange the letters.

S̲hape a sentence.

T̲ry combinations.

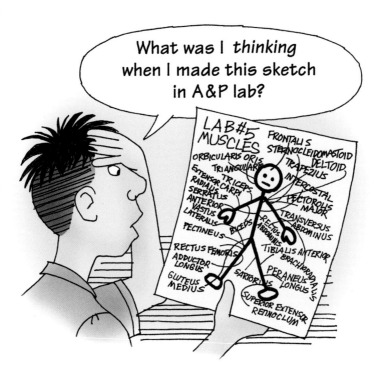

PART 2

Anatomy and Physiology Quick Reference

When you're on safari, among your most valuable tools are your *field guides*. Field guides are handy pocket references that help you quickly identify plants, animals, minerals, stars, and other natural features you see on your safari. Each guide may include labeled illustrations or photographs, range maps of where a particular feature is likely to be found, and checklists to keep track of what you've seen.

This **Anatomy and Physiology (A&P) Quick Reference** is a brief field guide to the human body that lays out the essential anatomic maps, functional diagrams, and summary tables needed for a basic understanding of human structure and function. We begin in Chapter 1 with some of the basic lingo you'll need: the stuff the body is made of, anatomic directions, names of body parts and systems, and a rough idea of how the body stays balanced. In later chapters we'll find maps and lists that will help us explore each of the major territories of the body. These tools will help bring topics into focus and clarify difficult concepts.

The **A&P Quick Reference** is organized into major themes covered in a typical human A&P course. They may be in a slightly different order than in your textbook—but you will have no difficulty finding them. Where appropriate, analogies and other learning aids that help illustrate complex topics are briefly outlined (boxed notes called *Field Notes*).

Field Notes

Using Models and Analogies

Professional scientists use models and analogies all the time to explain complex concepts; therefore it's no wonder that models and analogies are used so often in teaching about A&P—they work!

A **model** is a simplified version or description of something. For example, a model airplane is a simpler version of an airplane. It's a lot smaller than the real airplane and has far fewer parts and details

Continued

Field Notes—cont'd

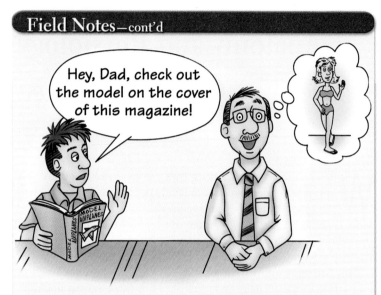

than the real airplane. However, a model airplane can teach you a great deal about the real airplane—especially if you've never seen it before. Therefore even though in many respects the model is not at all like the real airplane, it's similar enough to learn something about the real airplane. Likewise when a scientist talks about the lock-and-key model of enzyme action, you can imagine that the enzyme molecule acts like a key in a lock when it interacts with a specific molecule to either break it apart (unlock it) or to put it together with another molecule (lock it up). An enzyme isn't really a key, but the model of a key in a lock works to demonstrate how enzymes really do work.

An **analogy** compares something with which you're familiar to something with which you're not familiar in order to explain it. It really is a way of using something as a model that probably doesn't

Field Notes—cont'd

seem to resemble the real thing at first glance. For example, going to school is like driving a car. As with driving, schoolwork requires that you "stay on the road" and don't stray off the road defined by your learning objectives. As with driving, if you go too fast or too slow (or become distracted) you will not be able to keep up with "traffic" (the pace of learning in your course). Thus the idea of driving a car becomes a way for us to understand schoolwork in a different way.

In science we often use analogies to help explain how something works. For example, parts of the immune system act like the military. There is nonspecific (innate) immunity that includes many general strategies that you would use against any invader. In the military, that could be bullets from your gun, defensive walls, and alarms that sound if there's an attack. In the body, it includes your defensive skin, mucous membranes, phagocytic cells that gobble up invading particles, and chemicals that are released to sound an alarm in your body. Specific (acquired) immunity occurs when we develop specific mechanisms to combat specific invaders. In the military we may develop special artillery to use against the armor of a specific enemy or use a unique plan of attack with an enemy that is not susceptible to more common forms of attack. Actually this analogy has many elements of similarity—perhaps you can think of some yourself.

The great thing about analogies is that because they are familiar and different from the new concept that we are trying to learn, they make it easy to remember the various elements of the new concept—how it works in a simplified way.

This book uses the analogy of a safari—a voyage of discovery—to describe some successful ways to study A&P. We don't really come across any wild animals or swamps or thick jungles in our course, but the analogy is useful to learn some "survival skills" that will really help us in our course.

CHAPTER ONE

The Body as a Whole

TOPICS

Biochemistry, cell biology, tissues, body plan, homeostasis

Table 1-1	Units of Size		
UNIT	**SYMBOL**	**EQUAL TO**	**USED TO MEASURE**
Centimeter	cm	1/100 m	Objects visible to the eye
Millimeter	mm	1/10 cm	Very large cells, groups of cells
Micrometer (micron)	µm	1/1000 mm	Most cells, large organelles
Nanometer	nm	1/1000 µm	Small organelles, large biomolecules
Angstrom	Å	1/10 nm	Molecules, atoms

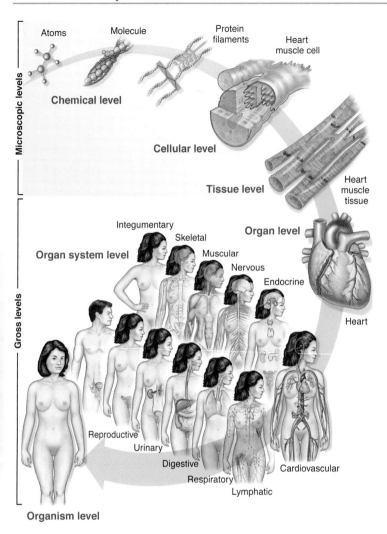

Atoms Molecule Protein filaments Heart muscle cell

Chemical level

Cellular level

Tissue level

Heart muscle tissue

Organ level

Integumentary

Skeletal

Organ system level Muscular

Nervous

Endocrine

Heart

Reproductive

Urinary

Digestive

Respiratory

Lymphatic

Cardiovascular

Organism level

Microscopic levels

Gross levels

Figure 1-1 Levels of organization. The smallest parts of the body are the atoms that make up the chemicals, or molecules, of the body. Molecules, in turn, make up microscopic parts called *organelles* that fit together to form each cell of the body. Groups of similar cells are called *tissues*, which combine with other tissues to form individual organs. Groups of organs that work together are called *systems*. All the systems of the body together make up an individual organism. Knowledge of the different levels of organization will help you understand the basic concepts of human A&P.

Table 1-2   Examples of Important Biomolecules

MACROMOLECULE	SUBUNIT	FUNCTION	EXAMPLE
Carbohydrates			
Glucose	Carbon, hydrogen, oxygen	Stores energy	Blood glucose
Ribose	Simple sugar (pentose)	Important in expression of hereditary information	Component of ribonucleic acid (RNA)
Glycogen	Glucose	Stores energy	Liver glycogen
Lipids			
Triglycerides	Glycerol + three fatty acids	Store energy	Body fat
Phospholipids	Glycerol + phosphate + two fatty acids	Make up cell membranes	Plasma membrane of cell
Steroids	Steroid nucleus (four-carbon ring)	Make up cell membranes Hormone synthesis	Cholesterol, various steroid hormones Estrogen
Prostaglandins	20 carbon unsaturated fatty acid containing five-carbon ring	Regulate hormone action; enhance immune system; affect inflammatory response	Prostaglandin E, prostaglandin A
Proteins			
Functional	Amino acids	Regulate chemical reactions	Hemoglobin, antibodies, enzymes
Structural	Amino acids	Component of body support tissues	Muscle filaments, tendons, ligaments

Table 1-2 Examples of Important Biomolecules—cont'd

MACROMOLECULE	SUBUNIT	FUNCTION	EXAMPLE
Nucleic Acids			
Deoxyribonucleic acid (DNA)	Nucleotides (sugar, phosphate, base)	Helps code hereditary information	Chromatin, chromosomes
RNA	Nucleotides (sugar, phosphate, base)	Helps decode hereditary infomation; acts as "RNA enzyme"; silencing of gene expression	Transfer RNA (tRNA), messenger RNA (mRNA), double-strand RNA (dsRNA)
Nucleotides and Related Molecules			
Adenosine triphosphate (ATP)	Phosphorylated nucleotide (adenine + ribose + three phosphates)	Transfers energy from fuel molecules to working molecules	ATP present in every cell of the body
Creatine phosphate (CP)	Amino acid + phosphate	Transfers energy from fuel to ATP	CP present in muscle fiber as "backup" to ATP
Nicotinic adenine dinucleotide (NAD)	Combination of two ribonucleotides	Acts as coenzyme to transfer high-energy particles from one chemical process to another	NAD present in every cell of the body
Combined or Altered Forms			
Glycoproteins	Large proteins with small carbohydrate groups attached	Similar to functional proteins	Some hormones, antibodies, enzymes, cell membrane components
Proteoglycans	Large polysaccharides with small polypeptide chains attached	Lubrication; increases thickness of fluid	Component of mucous fluid and many tissue fluids in the body

Continued

Table 1-2 Examples of Important Biomolecules—cont'd

MACROMOLECULE	SUBUNIT	FUNCTION	EXAMPLE
Lipoproteins	Protein complex containing lipid groups	Transport lipids in the blood	LDLs (low-density lipoproteins); HDLs (high-density lipoproteins)
Glycolipids	Lipid molecule with attached carbohydrate group	Component of cell membranes	Component of membranes of nerve cells

Table 1-3 Major Functions of Human Protein Compounds

FUNCTION	EXAMPLE
Provide structure	Structural proteins include keratin of skin, hair, and nails; parts of cell membranes; tendons
Catalyze chemical reactions	Lactase (enzyme in intestinal digestive juice) catalyzes chemical reaction that changes lactose to glucose and galactose
Transport substances in blood	Proteins classified as albumins combine with fatty acids to transport them in form of lipoproteins
Communicate information to cells	Insulin, a protein hormone, serves as chemical message from islet cells of the pancreas to cells all over the body
Act as receptors	Binding sites of certain proteins on surfaces of cell membranes serve as receptors for insulin and various other hormones
Defend body against many harmful agents	Proteins called *antibodies* or *immunoglobulins* combine with various harmful agents to render them harmless
Provide energy	Proteins can be metabolized for energy

Table 1-4	Major Functions of Human Lipid Compounds

FUNCTION	EXAMPLE
Energy	Lipids can be stored and broken down later for energy; they yield more energy per unit of weight than carbohydrates or proteins.
Structure	Phospholipids and cholesterol are required components of cell membranes.
Vitamins	Fat-soluble vitamins: vitamin A forms retinal (necessary for night vision); vitamin D increases calcium uptake; vitamin E promotes wound healing; and vitamin K is required for the synthesis of blood-clotting proteins.
Protection	Fat surrounds and protects organs.
Insulation	Fat under the skin minimizes heat loss; fatty tissue (myelin) covers nerve cells and electrically insulates them.
Regulation	Steroid hormones regulate many physiologic processes. Examples: estrogen and testosterone responsible for many of the differences between females and males; prostaglandins help regulate inflammation and tissue repair.

Table 1-5	Comparison of Deoxyribonucleic Acid and Ribonucleic Acid Structure

	DEOXYRIBONUCLEIC ACID (DNA)	RIBONUCLEIC ACID (RNA)
Polynucleotide strands	Two	One or two
Sugar	Deoxyribose	Ribose
Base pairs	Adenine-thymine Guanine-cytosine	Adenine-uracil Guanine-cytosine

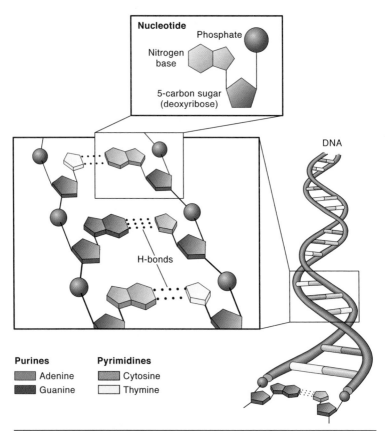

Figure 1-2 The deoxyribonucleic acid (DNA) molecule. Representation of DNA double helix showing the general structure of a nucleotide and the two kinds of "base pairs": adenine (*A, blue*) with thymine (*T, yellow*), and guanine (*G, purple*) with cytosine (*C, red*). Note that the G-C base pair has three hydrogen bonds and an A-T base pair has two. Hydrogen bonds are extremely important in maintaining the structure of this molecule.

Table 1-6	Summary of Protein Synthesis	
STEP	**LOCATION IN THE CELL**	**DESCRIPTION**
Transcription		
1	Nucleus	One region, or gene, of a deoxyribonucleic acid (DNA) molecule "unzips," exposing its bases.

Table 1-6   Summary of Protein Synthesis—cont'd

STEP	LOCATION IN THE CELL	DESCRIPTION
2	Nucleus	According to the principles of complementary base pairing, ribonucleic acid (RNA) nucleotides already present in the nucleoplasm temporarily attach themselves to the exposed bases along one side of the DNA molecule.
3	Nucleus	As RNA nucleotides align themselves along the DNA strand, they bind to each other and thus form a chainlike strand called *messenger RNA* (mRNA). This binding of RNA nucleotides is controlled by the enzyme RNA polymerase.

Preparation of the mRNA

STEP	LOCATION IN THE CELL	DESCRIPTION
4	Nucleus	As the preliminary mRNA strand is formed, it peels away from the DNA strand. This mRNA strand is a copy or *transcript* of a gene.
5	Nucleus	The spliceosome edits the mRNA molecule by removing noncoding portions of the strand (introns) and splicing the remaining pieces (exons).
6	Nuclear pores	Edited mRNA strand is transported out of the nucleus through the pores in the nuclear envelope.

Translation

STEP	LOCATION IN THE CELL	DESCRIPTION
7	Cytoplasm	Two subunits sandwich the end of the mRNA molecule to form a ribosome.
8	Cytoplasm	Specific transfer RNA (tRNA) molecules bring specific amino acids into place at the ribosome, which acts as a sort of "holder" for the mRNA strand and tRNA molecules. The kind of tRNA (and thus the kind of amino acid) that moves into position is determined by complementary base pairing: each mRNA codon exposed at the ribosome site will only permit a tRNA with a complementary *anticodon* to attach.

Continued

Table 1-6   Summary of Protein Synthesis—cont'd

STEP	LOCATION IN THE CELL	DESCRIPTION
9	Cytoplasm	As each amino acid is brought into place at the ribosome, an enzyme in the ribosome binds it to the amino acid that arrived just before it. The chemical bonds formed, called *peptide bonds,* link the amino acids together to form a long chain called a *polypeptide.*
10	Cytoplasm	As the ribosome moves along the mRNA strand, more and more amino acids are added to the growing polypeptide chain in the sequence dictated by the mRNA codons. (Each codon represents a specific amino acid to be placed in the polypeptide chain.) When the ribosome reaches the end of the mRNA molecule, drops it off the end, separating into large and small subunits again. Often, enzymes later link two or more polypeptides together to form a whole protein molecule.

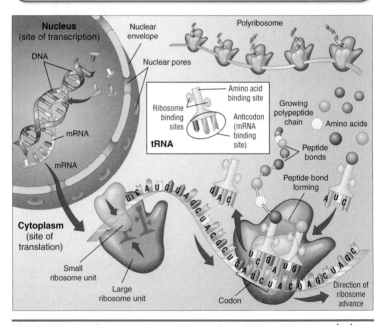

Figure 1-3 **Protein synthesis.** Protein synthesis begins with *transcription,* a process in which a messenger RNA (mRNA) molecule forms along one gene sequence of a deoxyribonucleic acid (DNA) molecule within the cell's nucleus.

Figure 1-3—cont'd As it is formed, the mRNA molecule separates from the DNA molecule, is edited, and leaves the nucleus through the large nuclear pores. Outside the nucleus, ribosome subunits attach to the beginning of the mRNA molecule and begin the process of *translation*. In translation, transfer RNA (tRNA) molecules bring specific amino acids—encoded by each mRNA codon—into place at the ribosome site. As the amino acids are brought into the proper sequence, they are joined together by peptide bonds to form long strands called *polypeptides*. Several polypeptide chains may be needed to make a complete protein molecule.

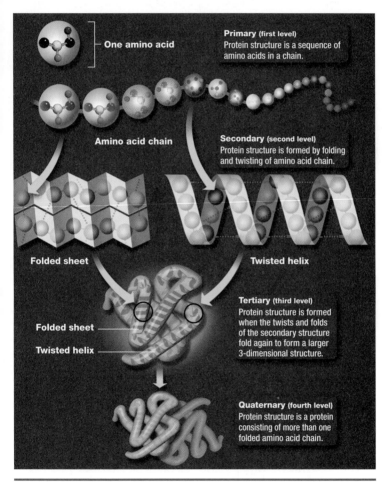

Primary (first level)
Protein structure is a sequence of amino acids in a chain.

One amino acid

Amino acid chain

Secondary (second level)
Protein structure is formed by folding and twisting of amino acid chain.

Folded sheet

Twisted helix

Tertiary (third level)
Protein structure is formed when the twists and folds of the secondary structure fold again to form a larger 3-dimensional structure.

Folded sheet

Twisted helix

Quaternary (fourth level)
Protein structure is a protein consisting of more than one folded amino acid chain.

Figure 1-4 Structural levels of protein. Primary structure: Determined by number, kind, and sequence of amino acids in the chain. **Secondary structure:** Hydrogen bonds stabilize folds or helical spirals. **Tertiary structure:** Globular shape maintained by strong (covalent) intramolecular bonding and by stabilizing hydrogen bonds. **Quaternary structure:** Results from bonding between more than one polypeptide unit.

Field Notes

Cooking Up Some Proteins

An often-used analogy to help us understand how proteins are synthesized in the cell is that of cooking. Of course, making proteins is not really the same as cooking up Grandma's carrot cake—but there are some useful similarities that help us understand the cellular processes. Use the accompanying table to follow this story of cooking that is really about making protein molecules.

You want to make carrot cake, so you go to your bookshelf (nucleus) where you keep your collection (genome) of cookbooks (DNAs). You find the recipe (gene) you want and make a photocopy of it (transcribe mRNA) so that you don't mess up the cookbook. Before leaving the bookcase (nucleus), you notice that Grandma wrote a bunch of stuff in the margins of the recipe that you don't really need. So you black out (edit) the stuff you don't need (introns), leaving the essential parts (exons) of the recipe (mRNA) intact.

You leave the bookcase (nucleus), go through the door (nuclear pore), and go to the kitchen (cytoplasm), where you put the recipe (edited mRNA) near the mixing bowl (rRNA). Next, you read (translate) the first word (codon) of the recipe (gene) and recognize the ingredient (specific amino acid), so you get it in its proper measuring cup (tRNA) and put it in the mixing bowl (rRNA). You read (translate) the next ingredient (amino acid) and get that kind of measuring cup (tRNA) to get that ingredient (specific amino acid) and put it into the mixing bowl (rRNA). Pretty soon you have a whole bunch of ingredients in the bowl (rRNA) that, after some mixing and baking, is a yummy carrot cake (polypeptide).

However, you like your carrot cake with cream cheese icing, so you go back to the cookbook collection (genome) and start the process again, this time using a different recipe (different gene) to make a different part of the dish (different polypeptide). When that's done (translated), you can put the icing on the cake, thereby finishing your favorite dessert (complete protein).

Acronym	Name	Cooking Analogy	Role in Cell Function
	Amino acid	Individual ingredient used to make a dish	A chemical group that links with other amino acids to form a polypeptide chain and eventually a whole protein

Field Notes—cont'd

Acronym	Name	Cooking Analogy	Role in Cell Function
	Codon	Word (in a recipe) that represents an individual ingredient; made up of any combination of 26 letters	Word (in a gene) that represents an individual amino acid; made up of any combination of four nucleotide bases
	Cytoplasm	The kitchen, where making a dish takes place	Area outside the nucleus where translation of proteins takes place
DNA	Deoxyribonucleic acid	The cookbook	The cell's "master copy" of the genetic code; a chromosome
	Editing	The process of blacking out un-needed parts of a copy of an individual recipe	The process of removing some segments of a gene (introns) in mRNA that are not needed for translation
	Exon	A part of the recipe copied from a cookbook that you need to make the dish	A part of the gene that remains after introns are removed; a part of a gene needed for translation
	Gene	Individual recipe (one of many recipes in a cookbook, or an individual copy of a recipe used in cooking)	Sequence of codons in DNA or RNA that codes for a specific amino acid
	Genome	Your entire collection of cookbooks, most of which are in a bookcase	The entire collection of DNA code, most of which is in the nucleus
	Intron	A part of the recipe copied from a cookbook that you don't really need to make the dish	A part of a gene that is removed from mRNA before it's translated into a protein

Continued

Field Notes—cont'd

Acronym	Name	Cooking Analogy	Role in Cell Function
mRNA	Messenger RNA	Individual recipe, copied from a cookbook, listing ingredients and the order in which they are added	Serves as working copy of one protein-coding gene
	Nucleus	Bookcase where you keep all your cookbooks	Cell structure containing most of the cell's genome
	Polypeptide strand	The actual dish that's made using a recipe, yet to be cut or folded or combined with another recipe	Product of protein synthesis, yet to be trimmed and folded and possibly combined with other polypeptides to form a whole protein
	Protein	The final, ready-to-serve form of a dish	The complete folded protein, ready to be used for any of many cell functions
rRNA	Ribosomal RNA	Mixing bowl into which the ingredients specified by a recipe are poured in the correct order	Component of the ribosome (along with proteins); attaches to RNA and participates in translation
snRNP	Small nuclear ribonucleoprotein	Black marking pen used to black out unneeded parts of an individual copy of a recipe	Component of the spliceosome; attaches to mRNA transcript to facilitate editing (removal of introns, splicing of exons) into final version of mRNA
	Transcription	The process of copying an individual recipe from a cookbook	The process of copying a gene from DNA to a strand of mRNA

Field Notes—cont'd

Acronym	Name	Cooking Analogy	Role in Cell Function
tRNA	Transfer RNA	Measuring cup that carries only one unit of an ingredient at a time and can only be used for one type of ingredient	Carries specific amino acid to a specific codon of mRNA at the ribosome during translation
	Translation	The process of reading a recipe, translating the instructions, and making the dish	The process of using genes on mRNA to construct a polypeptide chain on a ribosome

Table 1-7   Some Major Cell Structures and Their Functions

CELL STRUCTURE	FUNCTIONS
Membranous	
Plasma membrane	Serves as the boundary of the cell, maintaining its integrity; protein molecules embedded in plasma membrane perform various functions (e.g., serve as markers that identify cells of each individual, as receptor molecules for certain hormones and other molecules, and as transport mechanisms)
Endoplasmic reticulum (ER)	Ribosomes attached to rough ER synthesize proteins that leave cells via the Golgi apparatus; smooth ER synthesizes lipids incorporated in cell membranes, steroid hormones, and certain carbohydrates used to form glycoproteins—also removes and stores Ca^{++} from the cell's interior
Golgi apparatus	Synthesizes carbohydrate, combines it with protein, and packages the product as globules of glycoprotein
Lysosomes	Bags of digestive enzymes that break down defective cell parts and ingested particles; a cell's "digestive system"
Proteasomes	Hollow, protein cylinders that break down individual proteins that have been tagged by a chain of ubiquitin molecules
Peroxisomes	Contain enzymes that detoxify harmful substances

Continued

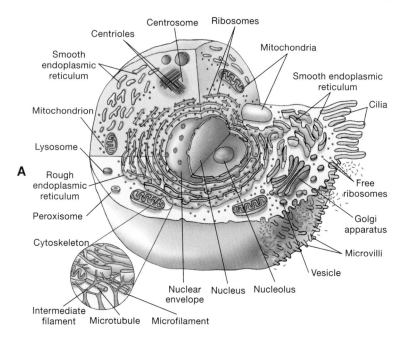

A

Centrioles
Centrosome   Ribosomes
Smooth endoplasmic reticulum
Mitochondria
Smooth endoplasmic reticulum
Mitochondrion
Cilia
Lysosome
Rough endoplasmic reticulum
Free ribosomes
Peroxisome
Golgi apparatus
Cytoskeleton
Microvilli
Vesicle
Nuclear envelope   Nucleus   Nucleolus
Intermediate filament   Microtubule   Microfilament

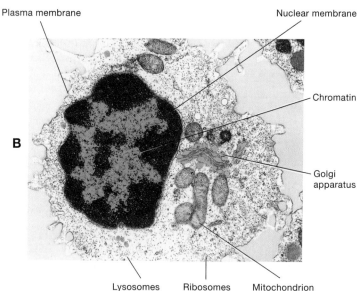

Plasma membrane
Nuclear membrane

B

Chromatin
Golgi apparatus
Lysosomes   Ribosomes   Mitochondrion

Figure 1-5 **Typical, or composite, cell. A,** Artist's interpretation of cell structure. **B,** Color-enhanced electron micrograph of a cell. Both show the many mitochondria, known as the *power plants of the cell.* Note, too, the innumerable dots bordering the endoplasmic reticulum. These are ribosomes, the cell's *protein factories.*

Table 1-7	Some Major Cell Structures and Their Functions—cont'd
CELL STRUCTURE	**FUNCTIONS**
Mitochondria	Catabolism; adenosine triphosphate (ATP) synthesis; a cell's "power plants"
Nucleus	Houses the genetic code, which in turn dictates protein synthesis, thereby playing essential role in other cell activities, namely, cell transport, metabolism, and growth
Nonmembranous	
Ribosomes	Site of protein synthesis; a cell's "protein factories"
Cytoskeleton	Acts as a framework to support the cell and its organelles; functions in cell movement; forms cell extensions (microvilli, cilia, flagella)
Cilia and flagella	Hairlike cell extensions that serve to move substances over the cell surface (cilia) or propel sperm cells (flagella)
Nucleolus	Part of the nucleus; plays an essential role in the formation of ribosomes

Field Notes

Drive a Cell Around the Block

When I visit my favorite car dealer, Al over at Subaru, he always wants me to take one of the new cars around the block to see how great it is. Well, it always is great because Al puts me in a car loaded with all kinds of cool options.

If I do decide to buy a car from Al, I probably won't get all those options. Some, like the fax machine, I really don't need. Others, like the racing wheels, are nice but I can't afford them. In addition, I'll probably ask for an extra option that wasn't on the car I test-drove—like all-weather floor mats because I'm a slob.

So why did Al put me in the car with all the options he knew I couldn't afford? Well, how would I know if I did want them if I'd never experienced them?

It's the same with the "generalized" or "typical" cell you see in most textbooks. First, remember it's a cartoon cell anyway, not a realistic image of a cell. Second, it's like the car that Al gave me to test drive—it has a lot of options you're not likely to see often all on one cell. However, when it comes time to study a type of cell

Continued

Field Notes—cont'd

with a particular option, you'll have already test-driven a cell with that option. In addition, every once in a while, you'll run across a cell that has a feature that wasn't in the typical cell you first studied. However, by then you'll be an expert on cell parts, and it won't phase you at all.

Table 1-8	Functional Anatomy of Cell Membranes

STRUCTURE		FUNCTION
Sheet (bilayer) of phospholipids stabilized by cholesterol	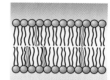	Maintains wholeness (integrity) of a cell or membranous organelle
Membrane proteins that act as channels or carriers of molecules	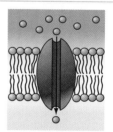	Controlled transport of water-soluble molecules from one compartment to another
Receptor molecules that trigger metabolic changes in membrane (or on other side of membrane)	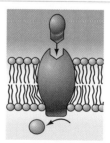	Sensitivity to hormones and other regulatory chemicals; involved in signal transduction

Table 1-8   Functional Anatomy of Cell Membranes—cont'd

STRUCTURE		FUNCTION
Enzyme molecules that catalyze specific chemical reactions	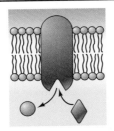	Regulation of metabolic reactions
Membrane proteins that bind to molecules outside the cell	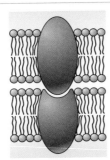	Form connections between one cell and another
Membrane proteins that bind to support	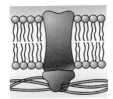	Support and maintain the shape of a cell or membranous organelle; participate in cell movement; bind to fibers of the extracellular matrix (ECM structures)
Glycoproteins or proteins in the membrane that act as markers	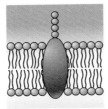	Recognition of cells or organelles

| Table 1-9 | Some Important Transport Processes |

PROCESS	DESCRIPTION
Passive	
Simple diffusion	Movement of particles through the phospholipid bilayer or through channels from an area of high concentration to an area of low concentration—that is, down the concentration gradient
Osmosis	Diffusion of water through a selectively permeable membrane in the presence of at least one impermeant solute (often involves both simple and channel-mediated diffusion)
Channel-mediated passive transport (facilitated diffusion)	Diffusion of particles through a membrane by means of channel structures in membrane
Carrier-mediated passive transport (facilitated diffusion)	Diffusion of particles through a membrane by means of carrier structures in membrane
Active	
Pumping	Movement of solute particles from an area of low concentration to an area of high concentration (up the concentration gradient) by means of an energy-consuming pump structure in the membrane

EXAMPLES

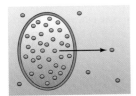

Movement of carbon dioxide out of all cells; movement of sodium ions into nerve cells as they conduct an impulse

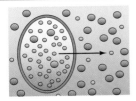

Diffusion of water molecules into and out of cells to correct imbalances in water concentration

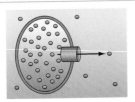

Diffusion of sodium ions into nerve cells during a nerve impulse

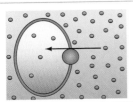

Diffusion of glucose molecules into most cells

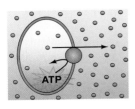

In muscle cells, pumping of nearly all calcium ions to special compartments—or out of the cell

Continued

Table 1-9   Some Important Transport Processes—cont'd

PROCESS	DESCRIPTION
Phagocytosis (endocytosis)	Movement of cells or other large particles into cell by trapping it in a section of plasma membrane that pinches off to form an intracellular vesicle; a type of *vesicle-mediated transport*
Pinocytosis (endocytosis)	Movement of fluid and dissolved molecules into a cell by trapping them in a section of plasma membrane that pinches off to form an intracellular vesicle; a type of *vesicle-mediated transport*
Exocytosis	Movement of proteins or other cell products out of the cell by fusing a secretory vesicle with the plasma membrane; a type of *vesicle-mediated transport*

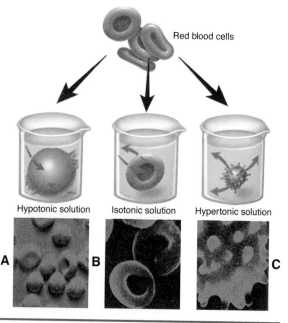

Figure 1-6 Effects of osmosis on cells.

EXAMPLES

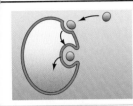

Trapping of bacterial cells by phagocytic white blood cells

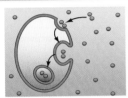

Trapping of large protein molecules by some body cells

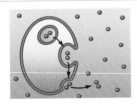

Secretion of the hormone, prolactin, by pituitary cells

Figure 1-6 Osmosis is the diffusion of water through a selectively permeable membrane. A, Normal red blood cells placed in a hypotonic solution may swell (as the *scanning electron micrograph* shows) or even burst (as the *drawing* shows). This change results from the inward diffusion of water (osmosis). **B,** Cells placed in an isotonic solution maintain a constant volume and pressure because the potential osmotic pressure of the intracellular fluid matches that of the extracellular fluid. **C,** Cells placed in a solution that is hypertonic to the intracellular fluid lose volume and pressure as water osmoses out of the cell and into the hypertonic solution. The "spikes" seen in the scanning electron micrograph are rigid microtubules of the cytoskeleton. These supports become visible as the cell "deflates." (Note: If the extracellular solution is hypotonic, then the cell is hypertonic to the solution; likewise if the solution is hypertonic, then the cell is hypotonic to the solution outside the cell.)

Field Notes

Fabric of the Body

I usually wear a sport coat in class when I'm teaching. Partly I do it because I want to look suave and sophisticated, but mostly I wear a jacket because that room is always cold, no matter what time of year.

The jacket is sort of like an organ of the body. It has its own distinct function but also works with my other clothes to keep me warm and stylish (just like an organ is part of a system and the whole organism).

Continued

Table 1-10   Major Tissues of the Body

TISSUE TYPE	STRUCTURE
Epithelial tissue	One or more layers of densely arranged cells with very little extracellular matrix (ECM); may form either sheets or glands
Connective tissue	Sparsely arranged cells surrounded by a large proportion of ECM often containing structural fibers (and sometimes mineral crystals)
Muscle tissue	Long fiberlike cells, sometimes branched, capable of pulling loads; extracellular fibers sometimes hold muscle fiber together
Nervous tissue	Mixture of many cell types including several types of neurons (conducting cells) and neuroglia (support cells)

Field Notes—cont'd

However, when you look at the jacket, you see that it's made up of several different fabrics. Each fabric has its own structure and function. The wool in the outer shell looks great and keeps me warm. The silky lining makes it easy to move around in. The thick padding in the shoulders makes me look even more macho than usual.

Likewise organs of the body are each made up of different tissues. Tissues are the fabrics of the body. Each tissue has its own structural and functional characteristics that contribute to the structure and function of the whole organ—and therefore the whole body.

FUNCTION	EXAMPLES IN BODY
Covers and protects body surface; lines body cavities; movement of substances (absorption, secretion, excretion); glandular activity	Outer layer of skin; lining of respiratory, digestive, urinary, reproductive tracts; glands of the body
Supports body structures; transports substances throughout the body	Bones, joint cartilage, tendons, and ligaments, blood, fat
Produces body movements; produces movements of organs such as stomach, heart; produces heat	Heart muscle; muscles of the head/neck, arms, legs, trunk; muscles in walls of hollow organs such as stomach, intestines
Communication between body parts; integration or regulation of body functions	Tissue of brain and spinal cord, nerves of the body, sensory organs of the body

Table 1-11 Components of the Extracellular Matrix (ECM)*

COMPONENT	EXAMPLE	DESCRIPTION
Water		Water molecules along with small number of ions (mostly Na^+ and Cl^-)
Proteins and glycoproteins	Collagen	Strong, flexible structural protein fiber
	Elastin	Flexible, elastic structural protein fiber
	Fibronectin	Rodlike glycoprotein
	Laminin	Glycoproteins arranged as a three-pronged fork
Proteoglycans	Various types	Protein backbone with attached chains of various polysaccharides: • Chondroitin sulfate • Heparin • Hyaluronate

*Not all components are present in all ECMs; examples include only some of the many major ECM components.

Table 1-12 Classification Scheme for Membranous Epithelial Tissues

SHAPE OF CELLS*	TISSUE TYPE
One Layer	
Squamous	Simple squamous
Cuboidal	Simple cuboidal
Columnar	Simple columnar
Pseudostratified columnar	Pseudostratified columnar
Several Layers	
Squamous	Stratified squamous
Cuboidal	Stratified cuboidal
Columnar	Stratified columnar
Varies	Transitional

*In the top layer (if more than one layer in the tissue).

FUNCTION	EXAMPLE OF LOCATION
Solvent for dissolved extracellular matrix (ECM) components; provides fluidity of ECM	All tissues of the body
Provides flexible strength to tissues	Tendons, ligaments, bones, cartilage, many tissues
Allows flexibility and elastic recoil of tissues	Skin, cartilage of ear, walls of arteries
Binds ECM to cells; communicates with cells through integrins	Many tissues of the body (e.g., connective tissues)
Binds ECM components together and to cells; communicates with cells through integrins	In basal lamina (basement membrane) of epithelial tissues
Shock absorber	Cartilage, bone, heart valves
Reduces blood clotting	Lining of some arteries
Thickens fluid; lubricates	Loose connective tissue, joint fluids

Table 1-13	Epithelial Tissues	
TISSUE	**LOCATION**	**FUNCTION**
Epithelial (Membranous)		
Simple squamous	Alveoli of lungs	Absorption by diffusion, filtration, osmosis
	Lining of blood and lymphatic vessels (called *endothelium;* classified as connective tissue by some histologists)	Absorption by diffusion of respiratory gases between alveolar air and blood
	Surface layer of pleura, pericardium, peritoneum (called *mesothelium;* classified as connective tissue by some histologists)	Absorption by diffusion and osmosis; also, secretion

Continued

Table 1-13	Epithelial Tissues—cont'd	
TISSUE	**LOCATION**	**FUNCTION**
Stratified squamous	Surface of mucous membrane lining mouth, esophagus, and vagina	Protection
	Surface of skin (epidermis)	Protection
Transitional	Surface of mucous membrane lining urinary bladder and ureters	Permits stretching
Simple columnar	Surface layer of mucous lining of stomach, intestines, and part of respiratory tract	Protection; secretion; absorption; moving of mucus (by ciliated columnar epithelium)
Pseudostratified columnar	Surface of mucous membrane lining trachea, large bronchi, nasal mucosa, and parts of male reproductive tract (epididymis and vas deferens); lines large ducts of some glands (e.g., parotid)	Protection
Simple cuboidal	Ducts and tubules of many organs, including exocrine glands and kidneys	Secretion, absorption
Stratified cuboidal or columnar	Ducts of sweat glands; lining of pharynx; covering portion of epiglottis; lining portions of male urethra	Protection
Epithelial (Glandular)		
	Glands	Secretion

Table 1-14	Connective Tissues	
TISSUE	**LOCATION**	**FUNCTION**
Fibrous		
Loose, ordinary (areolar)	Between other tissues and organs	Connection
	Superficial fascia	Connection
Adipose (fat)	Under skin; padding at various points	Protection, insulation, support, reserve food
Reticular	Inner framework of spleen, lymph nodes, bone marrow; filtration	Support
Dense Fibrous		
Irregular	Deep fascia	Connection
	Dermis	Support
	Scars	
	Capsule of kidney	
Regular	Tendons, ligaments, aponeuroses	Flexible but strong connection
	Walls of some arteries	Flexible, elastic support
Bone		
Compact bone	Skeleton (outer shell of bones)	Support, protection, calcium reservoir
Cancellous (spongy) bone	Skeleton (inside bones)	Support; provides framework for blood production
Cartilage		
Hyaline	Part of nasal septum; covering articular surfaces of bones; larynx; rings in trachea and bronchi	Firm but flexible support
Fibrocartilage	Disks between vertebrae, symphysis pubis	Firm but flexible support
Elastic	External ear, eustachian tube	Firm but flexible support
Blood	In the blood vessels	Transportation, protection

Table 1-15 Muscle and Nervous Tissues

TISSUE	LOCATION	FUNCTION
Muscle		
Skeletal (striated voluntary)	Muscles that attach to bones Extrinsic eyeball muscles Upper third of esophagus	Movement of bones Eye movements First part of swallowing
Smooth (nonstriated, involuntary, or visceral)	In walls of tubular viscera of digestive, respiratory, and genitourinary tracts In walls of blood vessels and large lymphatic vessels In ducts of glands	Movement of substances along respective tracts Change diameter of blood vessels, thereby aiding in regulation of blood pressure Movement of substances along ducts

Table 1-16 Membranes of the Body

TYPE	SUPERFICIAL LAYER	DEEP LAYER
Epithelial		
Cutaneous (skin)	Keratinized stratified squamous epithelium (epidermis)	Dense irregular fibrous connective tissue (dermis)
Serous	Simple squamous epithelium	Fibrous connective tissue
Mucous	Various type of epithelium	Fibrous connective tissue (lamina propria)
Connective		
Synovial	Dense fibrous connective tissue	Loose fibrous connective tissue

TISSUE	LOCATION	FUNCTION
Muscle—cont'd		
Smooth—cont'd	Intrinsic eye muscles (iris and ciliary body)	Change diameter of pupils and shape of lens
	Arrector muscles of hairs	Erection of hairs (gooseflesh)
Cardiac (striated involuntary)	Wall of heart	Contraction of heart
Nervous		
	Brain, spinal cord	Excitability, conduction, nerves

LOCATION	FLUID SECRETION	FUNCTION
Directly faces external environment	Sweat; sebum (skin oil)	Protection, sensation, thermoregulation
Lines body cavities that are not open to the external environment	Serous fluid	Lubrication
Lines tracts that open to the external environment	Mucus	Protection, lubrication
Lines joint cavities (in movable joints)	Synovial fluid	Helps hold joint together, lubricates, cushions

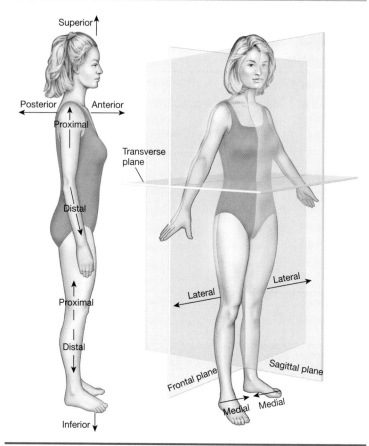

Figure 1-7 Directions and planes of the body. The transparent glasslike plates dividing the body into parts represent cuts or *sections* that can be made along a particular axis, or line of orientation, called a *plane*. There are three major **body planes** that lie at right angles to each other. They are called the *sagittal* (SA-jih-tul), *coronal* (kuh-RO-nul), and *transverse* (or *horizontal*) planes. Literally hundreds of sections can be made in each plane, and each section made is named after the particular plane along which it occurs. **Sagittal plane:** Lengthwise plane running from front to back is called a *sagittal plane*. Such a plane divides the body or any of its parts into right and left sides. If a sagittal section is made in the exact midline, resulting in equal and symmetrical right and left halves, the plane is called a *midsagittal plane*. **Coronal plane:** Lengthwise plane running from side to side; divides the body or any of its parts into anterior and posterior portions; also called a *frontal plane*. **Transverse plane:** Crosswise plane; divides the body or any of its parts into upper and lower parts; also called a *horizontal plane*. (Anatomic directions are listed in Table 1-17.)

Table 1-17	Anatomic Directions	
DIRECTIONAL TERM	**DEFINITION**	**EXAMPLE OF USE**
Left	To the left of the body (not *your* left, the subject's)	The stomach is to the *left* of the liver.
Right	To the right of the body or structure being studied	The *right* kidney is damaged.
Lateral	Toward the side; away from the midsagittal plane	The eyes are *lateral* to the nose.
Medial	Toward the midsagittal plane; away from the side	The eyes are *medial* to the ears.
Anterior	Toward the front of the body	The nose is on the *anterior* of the head.
Posterior	Toward the back (rear)	The heel is *posterior* to the head.
Superior	Toward the top of the body	The shoulders are *superior* to the hips.
Inferior	Toward the bottom of the body	The stomach is *inferior* to the heart.
Dorsal	Along (or toward) the vertebral surface of the body	Her scar is along the *dorsal* surface.
Ventral	Along (toward) the belly surface of the body	The navel is on the *ventral* surface.
Caudal	Toward the tail	The neck is *caudal* to the skull.
Cranial	Toward the head	The neck is *cranial* to the tail.
Proximal	Toward the trunk (describes relative position in a limb or other appendage)	The joint is *proximal* to the toenail.
Distal	Away from the trunk or point of attachment	The hand is *distal* to the elbow.
Visceral	Toward an internal organ; away from the outer wall (describes positions inside a body cavity)	This organ is covered with the *visceral* layer of the membrane.
Parietal	Toward the wall; away from the internal structures	The abdominal cavity is lined with the *parietal* peritoneal membrane.

Continued

Table 1-17 Anatomic Directions—cont'd

DIRECTIONAL TERM	DEFINITION	EXAMPLE OF USE
Deep	Toward the inside of a part; away from the surface (see *internal*)	The thigh muscles are *deep* to the skin.
Superficial	Toward the surface of a part; away from the inside (see *external*)	The skin is a *superficial* organ.
Internal	On the inside of a part (or the body)	The brain is an *internal* organ.
External	On the surface of a part, outside the part (or the body)	Hairs are *external* structures.
Medullary	Refers to an inner region, or medulla	The *medullary* portion contains nerve tissue.
Cortical	Refers to an outer region, or cortex	The *cortical* area produces hormones.
Ipsilateral	On the same side (of the body)	The left knee is *ipsilateral* to the left ankle.
Contralateral	On the opposite side of the body	The left knee is *contralateral* to the right knee.
Central	Toward the center of a part (or the body)	The *central* nervous system includes the brain and spinal cord.
Peripheral	Toward the outside boundary of a part (or the body)	Blood is pumped out of the heart and toward the *peripheral* vessels.
Basal	Toward or at the base of a part	The *basal* surface of the lung rests on the diaphragm.
Apical	Toward or at the point (apex) of a part	The *apical* surface of the cell possesses microvilli.

SPECIAL SECTION—THE ANATOMIC COMPASS

When I'm out on safari, I always have a map. I have to make sure the guide knows where he or she is going, right? The main reason I have it, though, is to learn the territory. We use maps of the body all the time in studying anatomy, too, to learn the territories of the body.

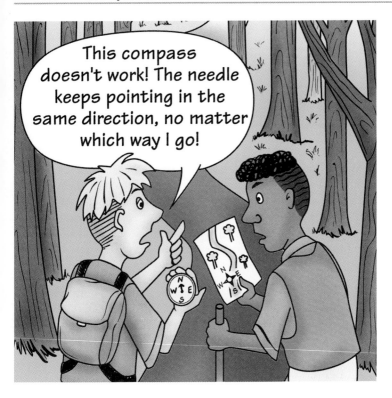

When I'm traveling in a new territory and look at a geographic map, I often don't know which way to hold it. However, that's easily corrected by looking at the little thing in the corner that looks like a compass face and has arrows marked N (north), S (south), E (east), and W (west). It's called a *rosette*—I guess because it looks kind of like a little rose. It tells me which way to look at the map and match the map features up with what I'm actually seeing.

To make the reading of anatomic figures a little easier, an *anatomic rosette* is used throughout this book (Figure 1-8). On many figures, you will notice a small compass rosette similar to those on geographic maps. Rather than being labeled N, S, E, and W, the anatomic rosette is labeled with abbreviated anatomic directions:

A	Anterior	**M**	Medial
D	Distal	**P** *(opposite A)*	Posterior
I	Inferior	**P** *(opposite D)*	Proximal
L *(opposite M)*	Lateral	**R**	Right
L *(opposite R)*	Left	**S**	Superior

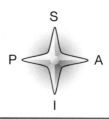

Figure 1-8 Anatomic rosette.

When I travel, it doesn't take long before I get somewhat familiar with the "lay of the land" and don't really need to check the rosette on the map anymore. It's the same with the anatomic rosette. At first, you may need to use it quite a bit to become oriented to a diagram, but after a while, you'll be so familiar with the body and its organs that you won't need it anymore.

Table 1-18	Body Systems		
FUNCTIONAL CATEGORY	**SYSTEM**	**PRINCIPAL ORGANS**	**PRIMARY FUNCTIONS**
Support and movement	Integumentary	Skin	Protection, temperature regulation, sensation
	Skeletal	Bones, ligaments	Support, protection, movement, mineral and fat storage, blood production
	Muscular	Skeletal muscles, tendons	Movement, posture, heat production
Communication, control, and integration	Nervous	Brain, spinal cord, nerves, sensory organs	Control, regulation, and coordination of other systems, sensation, memory
	Endocrine	Pituitary gland, adrenals, pancreas, thyroid, parathyroids, and other glands	Control and regulation of other systems

Table 1-18	Body Systems—cont'd		
FUNCTIONAL CATEGORY	**SYSTEM**	**PRINCIPAL ORGANS**	**PRIMARY FUNCTIONS**
Transportation and defense	Cardiovascular	Heart, arteries, veins, capillaries	Exchange and transport of materials
	Lymphatic	Lymph nodes, lymphatic vessels, spleen, thymus, tonsils	Immunity, fluid balance
Respiration, nutrition, and excretion	Respiratory	Lungs, bronchial tree, trachea, larynx, nasal cavity	Gas exchange, acid-base balance
	Digestive	Stomach, small and large intestines, esophagus, liver, mouth, pancreas	Breakdown and absorption of nutrients, elimination of waste
	Urinary	Kidneys, ureters, bladder, urethra	Excretion of waste, fluid and electrolyte balance, acid-base balance
Reproduction and development	Reproductive	*Male:* Testes, vas deferens, prostate, seminal vesicles, penis	Reproduction, continuity of genetic information, nurturing of offspring
		Female: Ovaries, fallopian tubes, uterus, vagina, breasts	

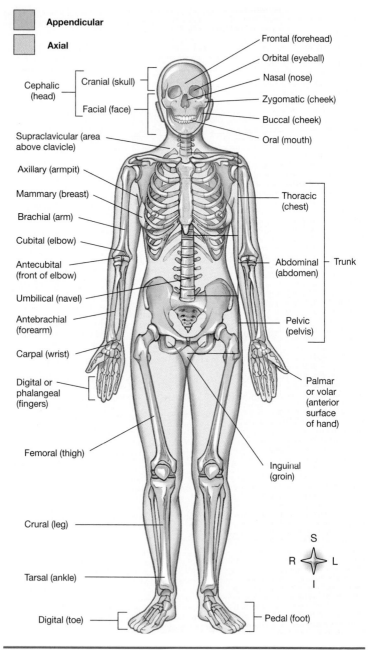

Figure 1-9 Specific body regions. Note that the body as a whole can be subdivided into two major portions: (1) axial (along the middle, or axis, of the body) and (2) appendicular (the arms and legs, or appendages). Names of specific body regions follow the Latin form, with the English equivalent in parentheses. Names are also listed in Table 1-19.

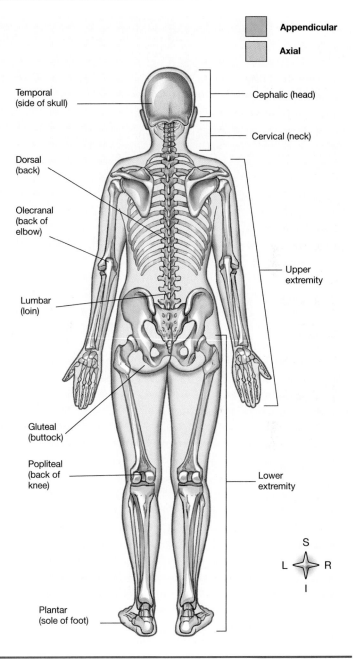

Figure 1-9—cont'd Specific body regions.

Table 1-19 Latin-Based Descriptive Terms for Body Regions*

BODY REGION	AREA OR EXAMPLE
Abdominal (ab-DOM-in-al)	Anterior torso below diaphragm
Acromial (ah-KRO-me-al)	Shoulder
Antebrachial (an-tee-BRAY-kee-al)	Forearm
Antecubital (an-tee-KYOO-bi-tal)	Depressed area just in front of elbow
Axillary (AK-si-lair-ee)	Armpit (axilla)
Brachial (BRAY-kee-al)	Upper arm
Buccal (BUK-al)	Cheek (inside)
Calcaneal (cal-CANE-ee-al)	Heel of foot
Carpal (KAR-pal)	Wrist
Cephalic (se-FAL-ik)	Head
Cervical (SER-vi-kal)	Neck
Coxal (COX-al)	Hip
Cranial (KRAY-nee-al)	Skull
Crural (KROOR-al)	Leg
Cubital (KYOO-bi-tal)	Elbow
Cutaneous (kyoo-TANE-ee-us)	Skin (or body surface)
Digital (DIJ-i-tal)	Fingers or toes
Dorsal (DOR-sal)	Back or top
Facial (FAY-shal)	Face
Femoral (FEM-or-al)	Thigh
Frontal (FRON-tal)	Forehead
Gluteal (GLOO-tee-al)	Buttock
Hallux (HAL-luks)	Great toe
Inguinal (ING-gwi-nal)	Groin
Lumbar (LUM-bar)	Lower back between ribs and pelvis
Mammary (MAM-er-ee)	Breast

*The left column lists English adjectives based on Latin terms that describe the body parts listed in English in the right column.

Table 1-19 — Latin-Based Descriptive Terms for Body Regions—cont'd

BODY REGION	AREA OR EXAMPLE
Manual (MAN-yoo-al)	Hand
Mental (MEN-tal)	Chin
Nasal (NAY-zal)	Nose
Navel (NAY-val)	Area around navel, or umbilicus
Occipital (ok-SIP-i-tal)	Back of lower skull
Olecranal (o-LECK-ra-nal)	Back of elbow
Oral (OR-al)	Mouth
Orbital or ophthalmic (OR-bi-tal or op-THAL-mik)	Eyes
Otic (O-tick)	Ear
Palmar (PAHL-mar)	Palm of hand
Patellar (pa-TELL-er)	Front of knee
Pedal (PED-al)	Foot
Pelvic (PEL-vik)	Lower portion of torso
Perineal (pair-i-NEE-al)	Area (perineum) between anus and genitals
Plantar (PLAN-tar)	Sole of foot
Pollex (POL-ex)	Thumb
Popliteal (pop-li-TEE-al)	Area behind knee
Pubic (PYOO-bik)	Pubis
Supraclavicular (soo-pra-cla-VIK-yoo-lar)	Area above clavicle
Sural (SUR-al)	Calf
Tarsal (TAR-sal)	Ankle
Temporal (TEM-por-al)	Side of skull
Thoracic (tho-RAS-ik)	Chest
Zygomatic (zye-go-MAT-ik)	Cheek

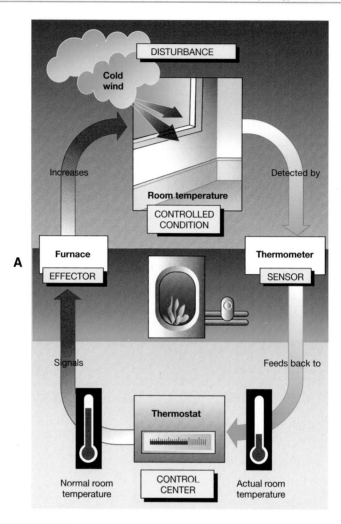

Figure 1-10 Basic components of homeostatic control mechanisms.
A, Heat regulation by a furnace controlled by a thermostat.

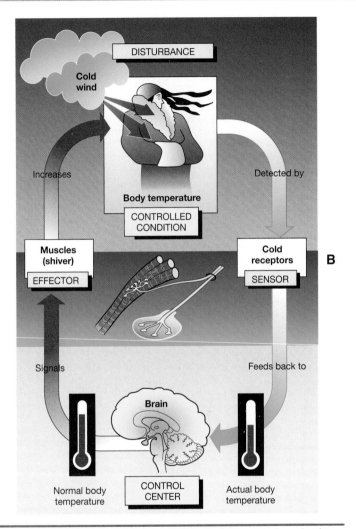

Figure 1-10—cont'd **Basic components of homeostatic control mechanisms.**
B, Homeostasis of body temperature. Note that in both examples **A** and **B,** a
stimulus or disturbance (drop in temperature) activates a sensor mechanism
(thermostat or body temperature receptor) that sends input to an integrating
(or control) center (on-off switch or hypothalamus), which then sends input
to an effector mechanism (furnace or contracting muscle). The resulting
heat that is produced maintains the temperature in a "normal range."
Feedback of effector activity to the sensor mechanism completes the
control loop.

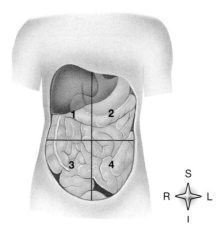

Figure 1-11 Division of the abdomen into four quadrants. Physicians and other health professionals frequently divide the abdomen into four quadrants to describe the site of abdominopelvic pain or locate some type of internal pathology such as a tumor or abscess. A horizontal and vertical line passing through the umbilicus (navel) divides the abdomen into right and left upper quadrants and right and left lower quadrants.

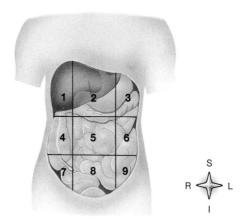

Figure 1-12 Nine regions of the abdominopelvic cavity. For convenience in locating abdominal organs, anatomists divide the abdomen like a tic-tac-toe grid into nine imaginary regions. Only the most superficial structures of the internal organs are shown here.

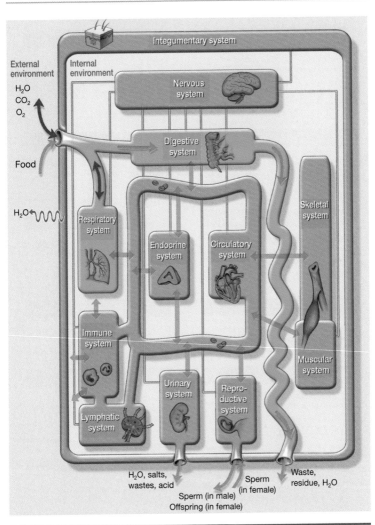

Figure 1-13 Diagram of the body's internal environment. The human body is like a bag of fluid separated from the external environment. Tubes, such as the digestive tract and respiratory tract, bring the external environment to deeper parts of the bag where substances may be absorbed into the internal fluid environment or excreted into the external environment. All of the "accessories" somehow help maintain a constant environment inside the bag, allowing the cells that live there to survive.

Continued

Integumentary system

Separates internal environment from external environment.

Nervous system

Major regulatory system of the internal environment: senses changes, integrates, and sends signals to effectors (muscular organs, glands).

Digestive system

Breaks down nutrients from the external environment and absorbs them into the internal environment.

Respiratory system

Exchanges O_2 and CO_2 between the internal and external environment.

Endocrine system

Regulates internal environment by secreting hormones that travel through the bloodstream to target areas.

Circulatory system

Transports nutrients, water, oxygen, hormones, wastes, and other materials within the internal environment.

Skeletal system

Supports, protects, and moves body. Also stores minerals.

Muscular system

Powers and directs skeletal movement.

Reproductive system

Produces sex cells that form off-spring, ensuring survival of genes. Female system is also site of fertilization and early development.

Urinary system

Adjusts internal environment by excreting excess water, salt, and other substances.

Immune system

Defends internal environment against injury from foreign cells and other irritants.

Lymphatic system

Drains excess fluid from tissues, cleans it, and returns it to the blood.

Figure 1-13—cont'd **Diagram of the body's internal environment.**

Field Notes

Wallenda Model

My friend, Tino, has an interesting job. He and his wife, Olinka (and most of his family), are in the circus. Performing as the "Flying Wallendas," Tino's family has amazed folks around the world with their ability to walk on the high wire. Tino is especially well known for his skill in walking on unusually high wires strung up over particularly high and hazardous areas—like across a waterfall or between skyscrapers. Yikes.

The image of a high-wire artist such as Tino Wallenda is a good model for understanding homeostasis in the body—what I call the *Wallenda Model.*

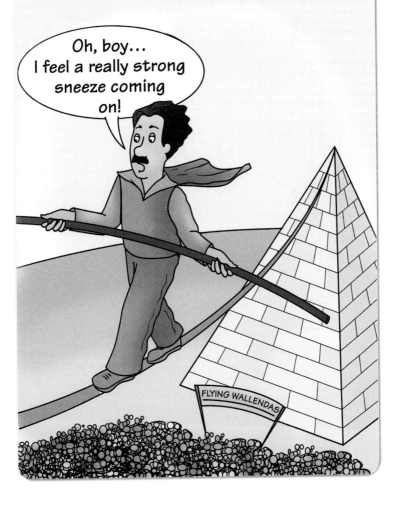

Field Notes—cont'd

Homeostasis is a kind of relative constancy of the body that is analogous to the kind of relative constancy of position that Tino must maintain on the high wire—if he is to survive.

Tino's grandfather, Karl, didn't survive. Karl was walking on a wire between two hotels in very windy conditions several decades ago. As good as Karl was, he couldn't maintain his position on the wire and fell to his death. I'm not telling you this to be morbid, but that's part of the usefulness of the model—if you don't maintain homeostatic balance in your body, you'll die. As a matter of fact, that's usually the mechanism involved in a person's death.

When Tino is on the high wire, the position just over the wire is his setpoint. If his "sensors" such as his eyes (vision receptors), ears (equilibrium receptors), and muscles (stretch receptors) tell him he's falling to his left, then the integrators in his brain will instruct his muscles to pull him a little to the right. This is a form of negative feedback—Tino's body is using feedback sensory information to regulate effectors, his muscles, to change his direction back toward the setpoint.

When you watch Tino perform, you'll notice that he sways back and forth and back and forth somewhat unpredictably as he crosses the wire. Likewise, in the body, conditions are constantly being disturbed and feedback mechanisms are being pulled back toward their setpoints. Tino is relatively constant in his position over the wire, just as your body conditions are relatively constant; and it takes energy to keep your body's feedback mechanisms working, just as it takes a lot of energy to keep Tino on the wire.

Something for which the Wallenda family is well known is the pyramid. That's where they stack Wallenda family members, one on top of the other, to form a human pyramid on the high wire. I still can't believe their famous 7-person, 3-high pyramid—and I've seen it many times! Imagine how well coordinated each of them needs to be to maintain the pyramid. Likewise, each feedback loop in your body is interdependent on others. If one feedback loop gets messed up, then that's likely to lead to many other problems.

CHAPTER TWO

Support and Movement

TOPICS

Skin, skeletal system, joints, muscles

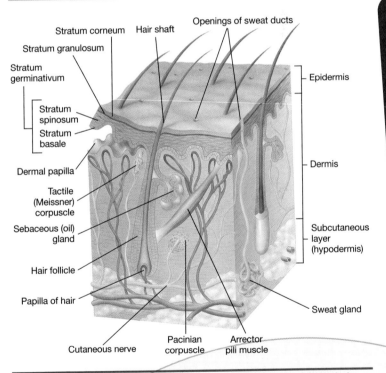

Figure 2-1 Diagram of skin structure. In this diagram the epidermis is raised at one corner to reveal the papillae of the dermis. (See Table 2-1 for details of skin structure.)

Table 2-1	Structure of the Skin

STRUCTURE	DESCRIPTION
Surface film	Thin film coating the skin; made up of mixture of sweat, sebum, desquamated cells/fragments, various chemicals; protects the skin
Epidermis	Superficial primary layer of the skin; made up entirely of keratinized stratified squamous epithelium; derived from the ectoderm; includes also hairs, sweat glands, sebaceous glands
Stratum corneum (horny layer)	Several layers of flakelike dead cells mostly made up of dense networks of *keratin* fibers cemented by *glycophospholipids* and forming a tough, waterproof barrier; the keratinized layer; possesses sulci (grooves) and friction ridges
Stratum lucidum (clear layer)	A few layers of squamous cells filled with *eleidin—* a keratin precursor that gives this layer a translucent quality (not visible in thin skin)
Stratum granulosum (granular layer)	Two to five layers of dying, somewhat flattened cells filled with dark staining keratohyalin granules and multilayered bodies of glycophospholipids; nuclei disappear in this layer
Stratum germinativum (growth layer)	General name for stratum spinosum and stratum basale together
Stratum spinosum (spiny layer)	Eight-to-ten layers of cells pulled by desmosomes into a spiny appearance
Stratum basale *(base layer)*	Single layer of mostly columnar cells capable of mitotic cell division; it's from this layer that all cells of superficial layers are derived; includes keratinocytes and some melanocytes
Dermal-epidermal junction	The basement membrane; a complex arrangement of adhesive components that glue the epidermis and dermis together
Dermis	Deep primary layer of the skin; made up of fibrous tissue; also includes some blood vessels, muscles, and nerves: derived from mesoderm
Papillary region	Loose fibrous tissue with collagenous and elastic fibers; forms nipplelike bumps (papillae); includes tactile corpuscles (touch receptors) and other sensory receptors

Table 2-1 Structure of the Skin—cont'd

STRUCTURE	DESCRIPTION
Reticular region	Tough network (reticulum) of collagenous dense irregular fibrous tissue (with some elastic fibers); forms most of the dermis
Hypodermis (subcutaneous layer, superficial fascia)	Loose, ordinary (areolar) connective tissue and adipose tissue; under the skin (not part of the skin); includes fibrous bands that connect the skin strongly to underlying structures; includes lamellar corpuscles (pressure receptors) and other sensory receptors

Table 2-2 Functions of the Skin

FUNCTION	EXAMPLE	MECHANISM
Protection	From microorganisms, dehydration, ultraviolet radiation, mechanical trauma	Surface film or mechanical barrier, keratin, melanin, tissue strength
Sensation	Pain, heat and cold, pressure, touch	Somatic sensory receptors
Permits movement and growth without injury	Body growth and change in body contours during movement	Elastic and recoil properties of skin and subcutaneous tissue
Endocrine	Vitamin-D production	Activation of precursor compound in skin cells by ultraviolet light
Excretion	Water, urea, ammonia, uric acid	Regulation of sweat volume and content
Immunity	Destruction of microorganisms and interaction with immune system cells (helper T cells)	Phagocytic cells, Langerhans' cells
Temperature regulation	Heat loss or retention	Regulation of blood flow to the skin and evaporation of sweat

Table 2-3	Bones of Skeleton (206 Total)*

AXIAL SKELETON (80 BONES TOTAL)

PART OF BODY	NAME OF BODY
Skull (28 bones total)	
Cranium (8 bones)	Frontal (1)
	Parietal (2)
	Temporal (2)
	Occipital (1)
	Sphenoid (1)
	Ethmoid (1)
Face (14 bones)	Nasal (2)
	Maxillary (2)
	Zygomatic (malar) (2)
	Mandible (1)
	Lacrimal (2)
	Palatine (2)
	Inferior nasal conchae (turbinates) (2)
	Vomer (1)
Ear bones (6 bones)	Malleus (hammer) (2)
	Incus (anvil) (2)
	Stapes (stirrup) (2)
Hyoid bone (1 bone total)	
Spinal column (26 bones total)	Cervical vertebrae (7)
	Thoracic vertebrae (12)
	Lumbar vertebrae (5)
	Sacrum (1)
	Coccyx (1)
Sternum and ribs (25 bones total)	Sternum (1)
	True ribs (14)
	False ribs (10)
Upper extremities (including shoulder girdle) (64 bones total)	Clavicle (2)
	Scapula (2)
	Humerus (2)
	Radius (2)
	Ulna (2)
	Carpals (16)
	Metacarpals (10)
	Phalanges (28)

Table 2-3	Bones of Skeleton (206 Total)*—cont'd

AXIAL SKELETON (80 BONES TOTAL)—cont'd

PART OF BODY	NAME OF BODY
Lower extremities (including hip girdle) (62 bones total)	Coxal (hip) (2)
	Fibula (2)
	Femur (2)
	Patella (2)
	Tibia (2)
	Tarsals (14)
	Metatarsals (10)
	Phalanges (28)

*An inconstant number of small, flat, round bones known as *sesamoid bones* (because of their resemblance to sesame seeds) are found in various tendons in which considerable pressure develops. Because the number of these bones varies greatly between individuals, only two of them, the patellae, have been counted among the 206 bones of the body. Generally two of them can be found in each thumb (in flexor tendon near metacarpophalangeal and interphalangeal joints) and great toe plus several others in the upper and lower extremities. *Wormian bones,* the small islets of bone frequently found in some of the cranial sutures, have not been counted in this list of 206 bones because of their variable occurrence.

Field Notes

Mountains, Hills, and Valleys

Imagine you're out on a trek through a wilderness unknown to you. You have your trusty cell phone and use it to occasionally call your friend who is familiar with the territory.

Let's say that your friend says, "Keep going north until you reach the Dardenne River." Therefore you trek onward, toward the north (you have your compass with you, of course). You reach a large rock outcropping and stop to call your friend. "I think I'm at the Dardenne River," you say, "What now?"

What's wrong with this picture? Obviously, you don't know a rock outcropping from a river—pretty bad if you're trekking by yourself in the wilderness!

It's the same when "trekking through" the human body ... you need to know your *hills* from *valleys* and *rivers* from *oceans*. Now I'm sure that you're already familiar with what a river is, but do you know what a *foramen* is? Or a *condyle?* What's the difference between a *condyle* and an *epicondyle?*

Continued

Field Notes—cont'd

If you look at Table 2-4, you'll see many of the different features you may find in the skeleton. If you learn that a foramen is a hole, it'll be pretty easy to find the *optic foramen*—it's a hole in the back of the eye socket for the optic nerve to pass. However, if you don't know what a foramen is, then you'll have to search your reference maps and descriptions—a much harder and less accurate way of doing it.

Most students don't take the time to become familiar with the terms in Table 2-4. Then they discover that finding all the assigned bone markings to be very difficult and time consuming. However, those students who familiarize themselves with the general types of features find it easy and fun to find the assigned bone markings.

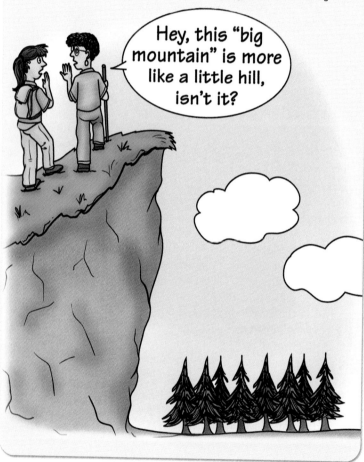

Table 2-4	Terms Used to Describe Bone Markings
TERM	**MEANING**
Angle	A corner
Body	The main portion of a bone
Condyle	Rounded bump; usually fits into a fossa on another bone, forming a joint
Crest	Moderately raised ridge; generally a site for muscle attachment
Epicondyle	Bump near a condyle; often gives the appearance of a "bump on a bump"; for muscle attachment
Facet	Flat surface that forms a joint with another facet or flat bone
Fissure	Long, cracklike hole for blood vessels and nerves
Foramen	Round hole for vessels and nerves (*pl.* foramina)
Fossa	Depression; often receives an articulating bone (*pl.* fossae)
Head	Distinct epiphysis on a long bone, separated from the shaft by a narrowed portion (or neck)
Line	Similar to a crest but not raised as much (is often rather faint)
Margin	Edge of a flat bone or flat portion of edge of a flat area
Meatus	Tubelike opening or channel
Neck	A narrowed portion, usually at the base of a head
Notch	A *V*-like depression in the margin or edge of a flat area
Process	A raised area or projection
Ramus	Curved portion of a bone, like a ram's horn (*pl.* rami)
Sinus	Cavity within a bone
Spine	Similar to a crest but raised more; a sharp, pointed process; for muscle attachment
Sulcus	Groove or elongated depression (*pl.* sulci)
Trochanter	Large bump for muscle attachment (larger than tubercle or tuberosity)
Tuberosity	Oblong, raised bump, usually for muscle attachment; small tuberosity is called a *tubercle*

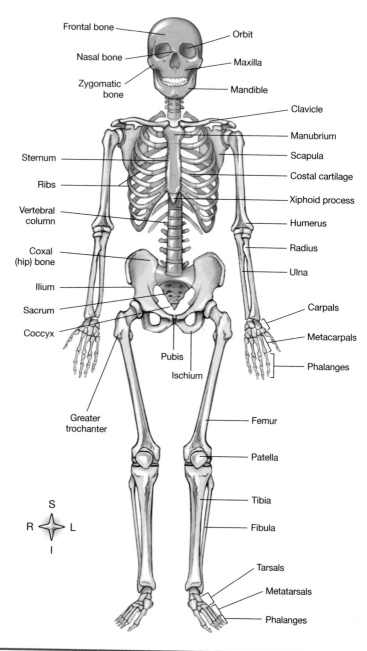

Figure 2-2 Skeleton. Anterior view.

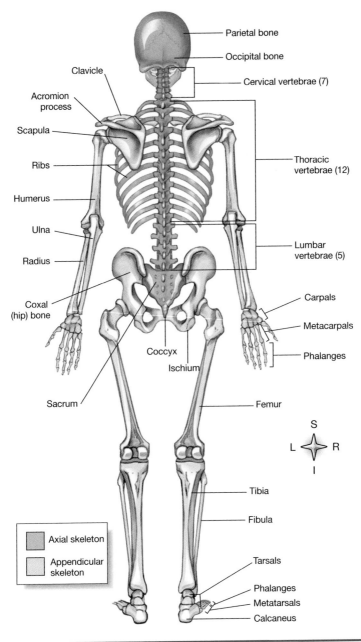

Figure 2-3 Skeleton. Posterior view.

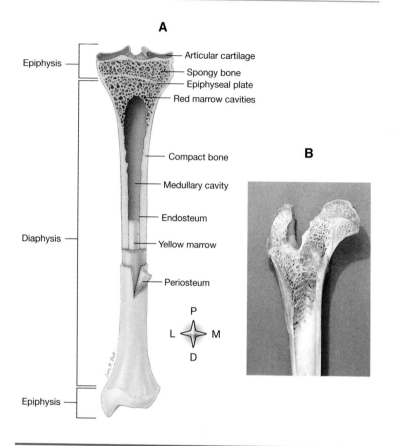

A

Epiphysis

Diaphysis

Epiphysis

- Articular cartilage
- Spongy bone
- Epiphyseal plate
- Red marrow cavities
- Compact bone
- Medullary cavity
- Endosteum
- Yellow marrow
- Periosteum

B

P
L ◇ M
D

Figure 2-4 Long bone. A, Longitudinal section of long bone (tibia) showing cancellous and compact bone. **B,** Cutaway section of a long bone.

PARTS OF A LONG BONE

Diaphysis—Main shaft of long bone

Epiphyses—Both ends of a long bone, made of cancellous bone filled with marrow

Articular cartilage—layer of hyaline cartilage that covers the articular surface of epiphyses

Periosteum—dense, white fibrous membrane that covers bone and attaches tendons firmly to bones

Medullary (or marrow) cavity—tubelike, hollow space in diaphysis; filled with yellow marrow in adult

Endosteum—thin epithelial membrane that lines medullary cavity

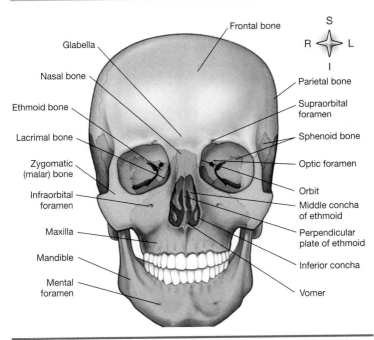

Figure 2-5 Anterior view of the skull. Contrast colors are added to the skull in this figure and in Figures 2-6 through 2-8 to distinguish more easily between the bones.

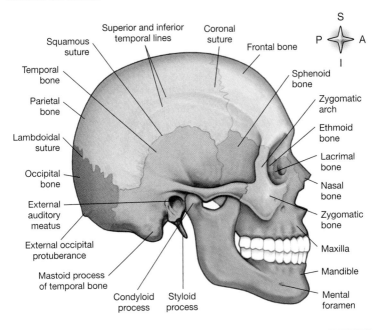

Figure 2-6 Skull viewed from the right side.

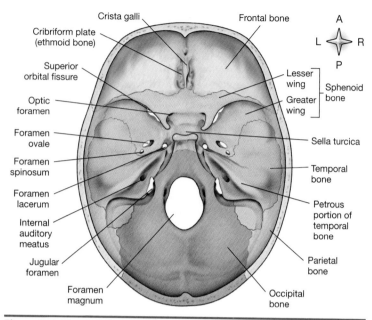

Figure 2-7 Floor of the cranial cavity. View is from above, with cap of skull removed.

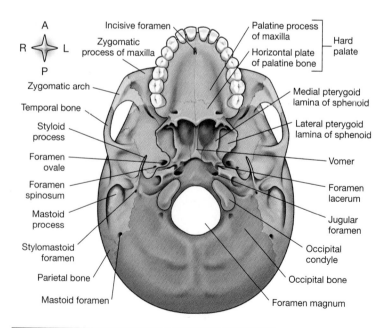

Figure 2-8 Skull viewed from below. Mandible has been removed.

Table 2-5 Cranial Bones and Their Markings

BONES AND MARKINGS	DESCRIPTION
Frontal	Forehead bone; also forms most of roof of orbits (eye sockets) and anterior part of cranial floor
Supraorbital margin	Arched ridge just below eyebrow, forms upper edge of orbit
Frontal sinuses	Cavities inside bone just above supraorbital margin; lined with mucosa; contain air
Frontal tuberosities	Bulge above each orbit; most prominent part of forehead
Superciliary ridges	Ridges caused by projection of frontal sinuses; eyebrows lie superficial to these ridges
Supraorbital foramen (sometimes notch)	Foramen or notch in supraorbital margin slightly medial to its midpoint; transmits supraorbital nerve and blood vessels
Glabella	Smooth area between superciliary ridges and above nose
Parietal	Prominent, bulging bones behind frontal bone; forms top sides of cranial cavity
Sphenoid	Keystone of cranial floor; forms its midportion; resembles bat with wings outstretched and legs extended downward posteriorly; lies behind and slightly above nose and throat; forms part of floor and sidewalls of orbit
Body	Hollow, cubelike central portion
Greater wings	Lateral projections from body, form part of outer wall of orbit
Lesser wings	Thin, triangular projections from upper part of sphenoid body; form posterior part of roof of orbit
Sella turcica (or Turk's saddle)	Saddle-shaped depression on upper surface of sphenoid body; contains pituitary gland
Sphenoid sinuses	Irregular mucosa-lined, air-filled spaces within central part of sphenoid
Pterygoid processes	Downward projections on either side where body and greater wing unite; comparable with extended legs of bat if entire bone is likened to this animal; form part of lateral nasal wall
Optic foramen	Opening into orbit at root of lesser wing; transmits optic nerve

Continued

| Table 2-5 | Cranial Bones and Their Markings—cont'd |

BONES AND MARKINGS	DESCRIPTION
Superior orbital fissure	Slitlike opening into orbit; lateral to optic foramen; transmits third, fourth, and part of fifth cranial nerves
Foramen rotundum	Opening in greater wing that transmits maxillary division of fifth cranial nerve
Foramen ovale	Opening in greater wing that transmits mandibular division of fifth cranial nerve
Foramen lacerum	Opening at the junction of the sphenoid, temporal, and occipital bones; transmits branch of the ascending pharyngeal artery
Foramen spinosum	Opening in greater wing that transmits the middle meningeal artery to supply meninges
Temporal	Form lower sides of cranium and part of cranial floor; contain middle- and inner-ear structures
Squamous portion	Thin, flaring upper part of bone
Mastoid portion	Rough-surfaced lower part of bone posterior to external auditory meatus
Petrous portion	Wedge-shaped process that forms part of center section of cranial floor between sphenoid and occipital bones; name derived from Greek word for stone because of extreme hardness of this process; houses middle and inner ear structures
Mastoid process	Protuberance just behind ear
Mastoid air cells	Mucosa-lined, air-filled spaces within mastoid process
External auditory meatus (or canal)	Tube extending into temporal bone from external ear opening to tympanic membrane
Zygomatic process	Projection that articulates with malar (or zygomatic) bone
Internal auditory meatus	Fairly large opening on posterior surface of petrous portion of bone; transmits eighth cranial nerve to inner ear and seventh cranial nerve on its way to facial structures
Mandibular fossa	Oval-shaped depression anterior to external auditory meatus; forms socket for condyle of mandible

Table 2-5	Cranial Bones and Their Markings—cont'd

BONES AND MARKINGS	DESCRIPTION
Styloid process	Slender spike of bone extending downward and forward from undersurface of bone anterior to mastoid process; often broken off in dry skull; several neck muscles and ligaments attach to styloid process
Stylomastoid foramen	Opening between styloid and mastoid processes where facial nerve emerges from cranial cavity
Jugular fossa	Depression on undersurface of petrous portion; dilated beginning of internal jugular vein lodged here
Jugular foramen	Opening in suture between petrous portion and occipital bone; transmits lateral sinus and ninth, tenth, and eleventh cranial nerves
Carotid canal (or foramen)	Channel in petrous portion; best seen from undersurface of skull; transmits internal carotid artery
Occipital	Forms posterior part of cranial floor and walls
Foramen magnum	Hole through which spinal cord enters cranial cavity
Condyles	Convex, oval processes on either side of foramen magnum; articulate with depressions on first cervical vertebra
External occipital protuberance	Prominent projection on posterior surface in midline short distance above foramen magnum; can be felt as definite bump
Superior nuchal line	Curved ridge extending laterally from external occipital protuberance
Inferior nuchal line	Less well-defined ridge paralleling superior nuchal line a short distance below it
Internal occipital protuberance	Projection in midline on inner surface of bone; grooves for lateral sinuses extend laterally from this process and one for sagittal sinus extends upward from it
Ethmoid	Complicated irregular bone that helps make up anterior portion of cranial floor, medial wall of orbits, upper parts of nasal septum, and sidewalls and part of nasal roof; lies anterior to sphenoid and posterior to nasal bones

Continued

Table 2-5 — Cranial Bones and Their Markings—cont'd

BONES AND MARKINGS	DESCRIPTION
Horizontal (cribriform) plate	Olfactory nerves pass through numerous holes in this plate
Crista galli	Meninges (membranes around the brain) attach to this process
Perpendicular plate	Forms upper part of nasal septum
Ethmoid sinuses	Honeycombed, mucosa-lined air spaces within lateral masses of bone
Superior and middle conchae (turbinates)	Help to form lateral walls of nose
Lateral masses	Compose sides of bone; contain many air spaces (ethmoid cells or sinuses); inner surface forms superior and middle conchae

Table 2-6 — Facial Bones and Their Markings

BONES AND MARKINGS	DESCRIPTION
Palatine	Form posterior part of hard palate, floor, and part of sidewalls of nasal cavity and floor of orbit
Horizontal plate	Joined to palatine processes of maxillae to complete part of hard palate
Mandible	Lower jawbone; largest, strongest bone of face
Body	Main part of bone; forms chin
Ramus	Process, one on either side, that projects upward from posterior part of body
Condyle (or head)	Part of each ramus that articulates with mandibular fossa of temporal bone
Neck	Constricted part just below condyles
Alveolar process	Teeth set into this arch
Mandibular foramen	Opening on inner surface of ramus; transmits nerves and vessels to lower teeth
Mental foramen	Opening on outer surface below space between two bicuspids; transmits terminal branches of nerves and vessels that enter bone through mandibular foramen; dentists inject anesthetics through these foramina

Table 2-6	Facial Bones and Their Markings—cont'd

BONES AND MARKINGS	DESCRIPTION
Coronoid process	Projection upward from anterior part of each ramus; temporal muscle inserts here
Angle	Juncture of posterior and inferior margins of ramus
Maxilla	Upper jaw bones; form part of floor of orbit, anterior part of roof of mouth, and floor of nose and part of sidewalls of nose

Table 2-7	Special Features of the Skull

FEATURE	DESCRIPTION
Sutures	Immovable joints between skull bones
Squamous	Line of articulation along top curved edge of temporal bone
Coronal	Joint between parietal bones and frontal bone
Lambdoidal	Joint between parietal bones and occipital bone
Sagittal	Joint between right and left parietal bones
Fontanels	"Soft spots" where ossification is incomplete at birth; allow some compression of skull during birth; also important in determining position of head before delivery; six such areas located at angles of parietal bones
Frontal (or anterior)	At intersection of sagittal and coronal sutures (juncture of parietal bones and frontal bone); diamond shaped; largest of fontanels; usually closed by $1\frac{1}{2}$ years of age
Occipital (or posterior)	At intersection of sagittal and lambdoidal sutures (juncture of parietal bones and occipital bone); triangular; usually closed by second month
Sphenoid (or anterolateral)	At juncture of frontal, parietal, temporal, and sphenoid bones
Mastoid (or posterolateral)	At juncture of parietal, occipital, and temporal bones; usually closed by 2 years of age
Air sinuses	Spaces, or cavities, within bones; those that communicate with nose called paranasal sinuses (frontal, sphenoidal, ethmoidal, and maxillary); mastoid cells communicate with middle ear rather than nose, therefore not included among paranasal sinuses

Continued

Table 2-7	Special Features of the Skull—cont'd

FEATURE	DESCRIPTION
Orbits Formed by	
Frontal	Roof of orbit
Ethmoid	Medial wall
Lacrimal	Medial wall
Sphenoid	Lateral wall
Zygomatic	Lateral wall
Maxillary	Floor
Palatine	Floor
Nasal Septum Formed by	
	Partition in midline of nasal cavity; separates cavity into right and left halves
Perpendicular plate of ethmoid bone	Forms upper part of septum
Vomer bone	Forms lower, posterior part
Cartilage	Forms anterior part
Wormian bones	Small islets of bone in sutures
Malleus, incus, stapes	Tiny bones, referred to as auditor ossicles, in middle ear cavity in temporal bones; resemble, respectively, miniature hammer, anvil, and stirrup

Table 2-8	Hyoid, Vertebrae, and Thoracic Bones and Their Markings

BONES AND MARKINGS	DESCRIPTION
Hyoid	U-shaped bone in neck between mandible and upper part of larynx; distinctive as only bone in body not forming a joint with any other bone; suspended by ligaments from styloid processes of temporal bones
Vertebral column	Not actually a column but a flexible, segmented curved rod; forms axis of body; head balanced above, ribs and viscera suspended in front, and lower extremities attached below; encloses spinal cord

Continued on page 117

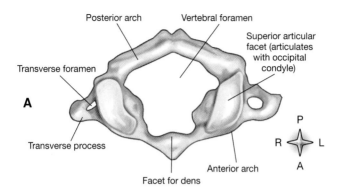

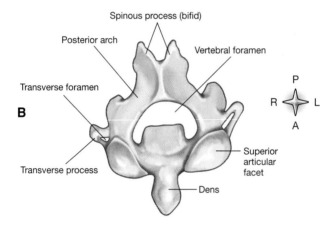

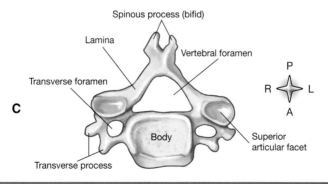

Figure 2-9 **Vertebrae. A,** Superior view of C1 (first cervical), the atlas. **B,** Superior view of C2 (second cervical), the axis. **C,** Superior view of C7 *(note the prominent spinous process).*

Continued

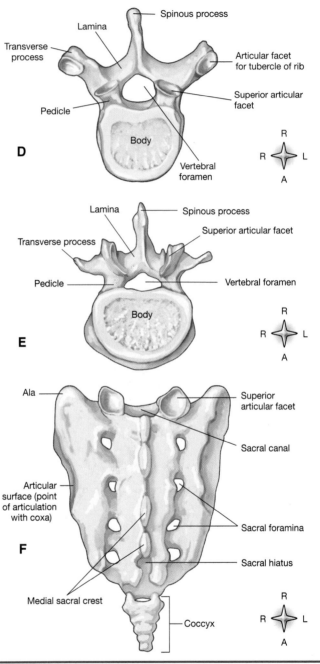

Figure 2-9—cont'd **Vertebrae. D,** Superior view of T10 (tenth thoracic). **E,** Superior view of L3 (third lumbar). **F,** Posterior view of the sacrum.

Table 2-8	Hyoid, Vertebrae, and Thoracic Bones and Their Markings—cont'd

BONES AND MARKINGS	DESCRIPTION
General features	Anterior part of each vertebra (except first two cervical) consists of body; posterior part of vertebrae consists of neural arch, which, in turn, consists of two pedicles, two laminae, and seven processes projecting from laminae
Body	Main part; flat, round mass located anteriorly; supporting or weight-bearing part of vertebra
Pedicles	Short projections extending posteriorly from body
Lamina	Posterior part of vertebra to which pedicles join and from which processes project
Neural arch	Formed by pedicles and laminae; protects spinal cord posteriorly; congenital absence of one or more neural arches is known as *spina bifida* (cord may protrude right through skin)
Spinous process	Sharp process projecting inferiorly from laminae in midline
Transverse processes	Right and left lateral projections from laminae
Superior articulating processes	Project upward from laminae
Inferior articulating processes	Project downward from laminae; articulate with superior articulating processes of vertebrae below
Spinal foramen	Hole in center of vertebra formed by union of body, pedicles, and laminae; spinal foramina, when vertebrae, superimposed one on the other, form spinal cavity that houses spinal cord
Intervertebral foramina	Opening between vertebrae through which spinal nerves emerge
Cervical vertebrae	First or upper seven vertebrae; foramen in each transverse process for transmission of vertebral artery, vein, and plexus of nerves; short bifurcated spinous processes except on seventh vertebra, where it's extra long and may be felt as protrusion when head bent forward; bodies of these vertebrae small, whereas spinal foramina large and triangular

Continued

Table 2-8	Hyoid, Vertebrae, and Thoracic Bones and Their Markings—cont'd

BONES AND MARKINGS	DESCRIPTION
Atlas	First cervical vertebra; lacks body and spinous process; superior articulating processes concave ovals that act as rockerlike cradles for condyles of occipital bone; named *atlas* because it supports the head as Atlas supports the world in Greek mythology
Axis (epistropheus)	Second cervical vertebra, so named because atlas rotates about this bone in rotating movements of head; dens, or odontoid process, peglike projection upward from body of axis, forming pivot for rotation of atlas
Thoracic vertebrae	Next 12 vertebrae; 12 pairs of ribs attached to these; stronger, with more massive bodies than cervical vertebrae; no transverse foramina; two sets of facets for articulations with corresponding rib: one on body, second on transverse process; upper thoracic vertebrae with elongated spinous process
Lumbar vertebrae	Next five vertebrae; strong, massive; superior articulating processes directed medially instead of upward; inferior articulating processes, laterally instead of downward; short, blunt spinous process
Sacrum	Five separate vertebrae until about 25 years of age; then fused to form one wedge-shaped bone
Sacral promontory	Protuberance from anterior, upper border of sacrum into pelvis; of obstetric importance because its size limits anteroposterior diameter of pelvic inlet
Coccyx	Four or five separate vertebrae in child but fused into one in adult
Curves	Curves have great structural importance because they increase carrying strength of vertebral column, make balance possible in upright position (if column were straight, weight of viscera would pull body forward), absorb jolts from walking (straight column would transmit jolts straight to head), and protect column from fracture

Table 2-8　　Hyoid, Vertebrae, and Thoracic Bones and Their Markings—cont'd

BONES AND MARKINGS	DESCRIPTION
Primary	Column curves at birth from head to sacrum with convexity posteriorly; after child stands, convexity persists only in *thoracic* and *sacral* regions, which therefore are called *primary curves*
Secondary	Concavities in *cervical* and *lumbar* regions; cervical concavity results from infant's attempts to hold head erect (2 to 4 months); lumbar concavity, from balancing efforts in learning to walk (10 to 18 months)
Sternum	Breastbone; flat, dagger-shaped bone; sternum, ribs, and thoracic vertebrae together form bony cage known as *thorax*
Body	Main central part of bone
Manubrium	Flaring, upper part
Xiphoid process	Projection of cartilage at lower border of bone
Ribs	
True ribs	Upper seven pairs; fasten to sternum by costal cartilages
False ribs	False ribs do not attach to sternum directly; upper three pairs of false ribs attach by means of costal cartilage of seventh ribs; last two pairs do not attach to sternum at all, therefore called floating ribs
Head	Projection at posterior end of rib; articulates with corresponding thoracic vertebra and one above, except last three pairs, which join corresponding vertebrae only
Neck	Constricted portion just below head
Tubercle	Small knob just below neck; articulates with transverse process of corresponding thoracic vertebra; missing in lowest three ribs
Body or shaft	Main part of rib
Costal cartilage	Cartilage at sternal end of true ribs; attaches ribs (except floating ribs) to sternum

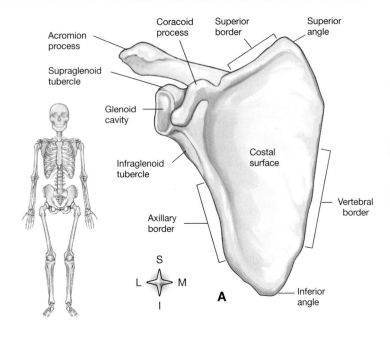

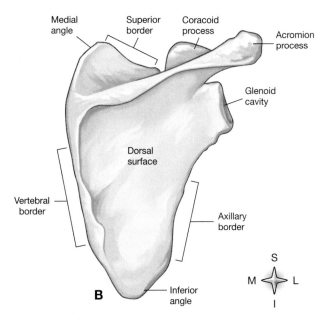

Figure 2-10 **Right scapula. A,** Anterior view. **B,** Posterior view. The small inset shows the relative position of the right scapula within the entire skeleton.

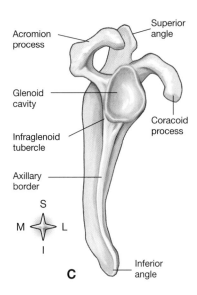

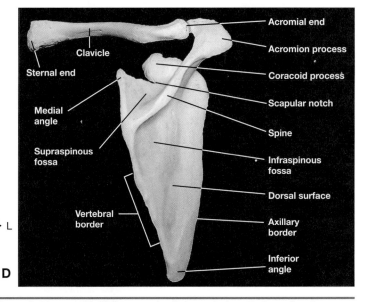

Figure 2-10—cont'd Right scapula. C, Lateral view. **D,** Posterior view showing articulation with clavicle.

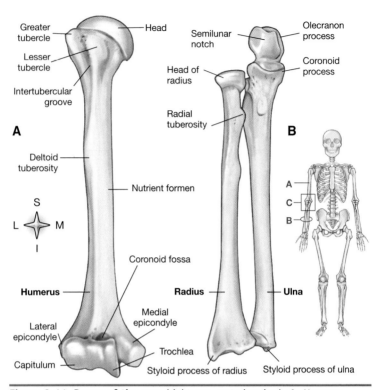

Figure 2-11 **Bones of the arm** (right arm, anterior view). **A,** Humerus (upper arm). **B,** Radius and ulna (forearm). The inset shows the relative position of the right arm bones within the entire skeleton.

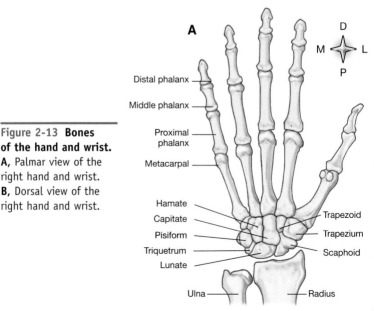

Figure 2-13 **Bones of the hand and wrist.** **A,** Palmar view of the right hand and wrist. **B,** Dorsal view of the right hand and wrist.

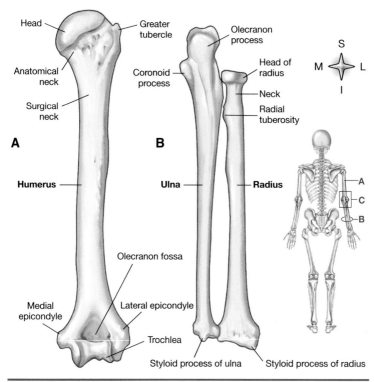

Figure 2-12 Bones of the arm *(right arm, posterior view)*. **A,** Humerus (upper arm). **B,** Radius and ulna *(forearm)*. The inset shows the relative position of the right arm bones within the entire skeleton.

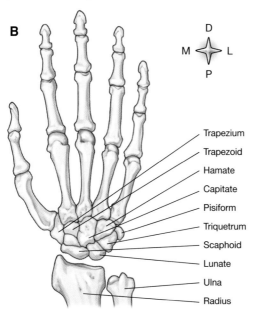

Table 2-9 — Upper Extremity Bones and Their Markings

BONES AND MARKINGS	DESCRIPTION
Clavicle	Collar bones; shoulder girdle joined to axial skeleton by articulation of clavicles with sternum (scapula does not form joint with axial skeleton)
Scapula	Shoulder blades; scapulae and clavicles together make up shoulder girdle

Borders
  Superior
  Vertebral
  Axillary
	
	Upper margin
	Margin toward vertebral column
	Lateral margin

Spine	Sharp ridge running diagonally across posterior surface of shoulder blade
Acromion process	Slightly flaring projection at lateral end of scapular spine; may be felt as tip of shoulder; articulates with clavicle
Coracoid process	Projection on anterior surface from upper border of bone; may be felt in groove between deltoid and pectoralis major muscles, about 1 inch below clavicle
Glenoid cavity	Arm socket
Humerus	Long bone of upper arm
Head	Smooth, hemispheric enlargement at proximal end of humerus
Anatomic neck	Oblique groove just below head
Greater tubercle	Rounded projection lateral to head on anterior surface
Lesser tubercle	Prominent projection on anterior surface just below anatomic neck
Intertubercular groove	Deep groove between greater and lesser tubercles; long tendon of biceps muscle lodges here
Surgical neck	Region just below tubercles; so named because of its liability to fracture
Deltoid tuberosity	V-shaped, rough area about midway down shaft where deltoid muscle inserts
Radial groove	Groove running obliquely downward from deltoid tuberosity; lodges radial nerve
Epicondyles (medial and lateral)	Rough projections at both sides of distal end
Capitulum	Rounded knob below lateral epicondyle; articulates with radius; sometimes called *radial head* of humerus

Table 2-9 — Upper Extremity Bones and Their Markings—cont'd

BONES AND MARKINGS	DESCRIPTION
Trochlea	Projection with deep depression through center similar to shape of pulley; articulates with ulna
Olecranon fossa	Depression on posterior surface just above trochlea; receives olecranon process of ulna when lower arm extends
Coronoid fossa	Depression on anterior surface above trochlea; receives coronoid process of ulna in flexion of lower arm
Radius	Bone of thumb side of forearm
Head	Disk-shaped process forming proximal end of radius; articulates with capitulum of humerus and with radial notch of ulna
Radial tuberosity	Roughened projection on ulnar side, short distance below head; biceps muscle inserts here
Styloid process	Protuberance at distal end on lateral surface (with forearm in anatomic position)
Ulna	Bone on little finger side of forearm; longer than radius
Olecranon process	Elbow
Coronoid process	Projection on anterior surface of proximal end of ulna; trochlea of humerus fits snugly between olecranon and coronoid processes
Semilunar notch	Curved notch between olecranon and coronoid process into which trochlea fits
Radial notch	Curved notch lateral and inferior to semilunar notch; head of radius fits into this concavity
Head	Rounded process at distal end; does not articulate with wrist bones but with fibrocartilaginous disk
Styloid process	Sharp protuberance at distal end; can be seen from outside on posterior surface
Carpals	Wrist bones; arranged in two rows at proximal end of hand; proximal row (from little finger toward thumb) —*pisiform, triquetrum, lunate,* and *scaphoid*; distal row—*hamate, capitate, trapezoid,* and *trapezium*
Metacarpals	Long bones forming framework of palm of hand; numbered I through V
Phalanges	Miniature long bones of fingers, three (proximal, middle, distal) in each finger, two (proximal, distal) in each thumb

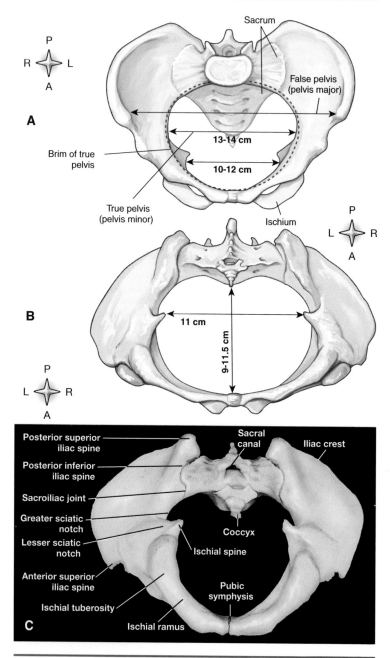

Figure 2-14 The female pelvis. A, Pelvis viewed from above. Note that the brim of the true pelvis *(dotted line)* marks the boundary between the superior false pelvis *(pelvis major)* and the inferior true pelvis *(pelvis minor).* **B** and **C,** Pelvis viewed from below. Comparison of the male and female pelvis is shown in Figure 2-18.

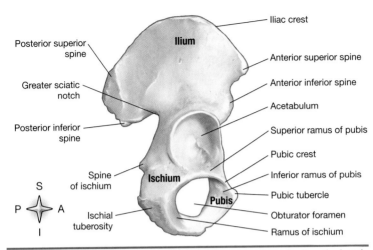

Figure 2-15 Right coxal (hip) bone. The right coxal bone is disarticulated from the bony pelvis and viewed from the side.

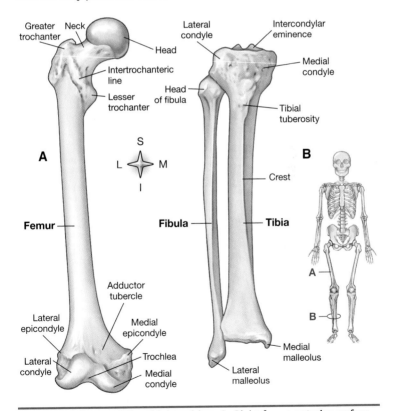

Figure 2-16 Bones of the thigh and leg. A, Right femur, anterior surface. **B,** Right tibia and fibula, anterior surface. The inset shows the relative position of the bones of the thigh and leg within the entire skeleton.

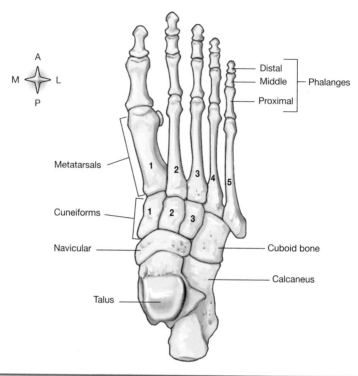

Figure 2-17 The foot. Bones of the right foot viewed from above. Tarsal bones consist of cuneiforms, navicular, talus, cuboid, and calcaneus.

Table 2-10	Lower Extremity Bones and Their Markings
BONES AND MARKINGS	**DESCRIPTION**
Coxal	Large hip bone; with sacrum and coccyx, forms basinlike pelvic cavity; lower extremities attached to axial skeleton by coxal bones
Ilium	Upper, flaring portion
Ischium	Lower, posterior portion
Pubic bone (pubis)	Medial, anterior section
Acetabulum	Hip socket; formed by union of ilium, ischium, and pubis

Table 2-10	Lower Extremity Bones and Their Markings—cont'd

BONES AND MARKINGS	DESCRIPTION
Iliac crests	Upper, curving boundary of ilium
Iliac spines	
Anterior superior	Prominent projection at anterior end of iliac crest; can be felt externally as "point" of hip
Anterior inferior	Less prominent projection short distance below anterior superior spine
Posterior superior	At posterior end of iliac crest
Posterior inferior	Just below posterior superior spine
Greater sciatic notch	Large notch on posterior surface of ilium just below posterior inferior spine
Ischial tuberosity	Large, rough, quadrilateral process forming inferior part of ischium; in erect sitting position, body rests on these tuberosities
Ischial spine	Pointed projection just above tuberosity
Symphysis pubis	Cartilaginous, amphiarthrotic joint between pubic bones
Superior ramus of pubis	Part of pubis lying between symphysis and acetabulum; forms upper part of obturator foramen
Inferior ramus	Part extending down from symphysis; unites with ischium
Pubic arch	Angle formed by two inferior rami
Pubic crest	Upper margin of superior ramus
Pubic tubercle	Rounded process at end of crest
Obturator foramen	Large hole in anterior surface of os coxae; formed by pubis and ischium; largest foramen in body
Pelvic brim (or inlet)	Boundary of aperture leading into true pelvis; formed by pubic crests, iliopectineal lines, and sacral promontory; size and shape of this inlet have obstetric importance, because if any of its diameters are too small, infant skull cannot enter true pelvis for natural birth
True pelvis (or pelvis minor)	Space below pelvic brim; true "basin" with bone and muscle walls and muscle floor; pelvic organs located in this space

Continued

Table 2-10	Lower Extremity Bones and Their Markings—cont'd

BONES AND MARKINGS	DESCRIPTION
False pelvis (or pelvis major)	Broad, shallow space above pelvic brim, or pelvic inlet; name "false pelvis" is misleading, because this space is actually part of abdominal cavity, not pelvic cavity
Pelvic outlet	Irregular circumference marking lower limits of true pelvis; bounded by tip of coccyx and two ischial tuberosities
Pelvic girdle (or bony pelvis)	Complete bony ring; composed of two hip bones (ossa coxae), sacrum, and coccyx; forms firm base by which trunk rests on thighs and for attachment of lower extremities to axial skeleton
Femur	Thigh bone; largest, strongest bone of body
Head	Rounded upper end of bone; fits into acetabulum
Neck	Constricted portion just below head
Greater trochanter	Protuberance located inferiorly and laterally to head
Lesser trochanter	Small protuberance located inferiorly and medially to greater trochanter
Intertrochanteric line	Line extending between greater and lesser trochanter
Linea aspera	Prominent ridge extending lengthwise along concave posterior surface
Supracondylar ridges	Two ridges formed by division of linea aspera at its lower end; medial supracondylar ridge extends inward to inner condyle, lateral ridge to outer condyle
Condyles	Large, rounded bulges at distal end of femur; one medial and one lateral
Epicondyles	Blunt projections from the sides of the condyles; one on the medial aspect and one on the lateral aspect
Adductor tubercle	Small projection just above medial condyle; marks termination of medial supracondylar ridge
Trochlea	Smooth depression between condyles on anterior surface; articulates with patella
Intercondyloid fossa (notch)	Deep depression between condyles on posterior surface; cruciate ligaments that help bind femur to tibia lodge in this notch

Table 2-10   Lower Extremity Bones and Their Markings—cont'd

BONES AND MARKINGS	DESCRIPTION
Patella	Kneecap; largest sesamoid bone of body; embedded in tendon of quadriceps femoris muscle
Tibia	Shin bone
Condyles	Bulging prominences at proximal end of tibia; upper surfaces concave for articulation with femur
Intercondylar eminence	Upward projection on articular surface between condyles
Crest	Sharp ridge on anterior surface
Tibial tuberosity	Projection in midline on anterior surface
Medial malleolus	Rounded downward projection at distal end of tibia; forms prominence on medial surface of ankle
Fibula	Long, slender bone of lateral side of lower leg
Lateral malleolus	Rounded prominence at distal end of fibula; forms prominence on lateral surface of ankle
Tarsals	Bones that form heel and proximal or posterior half of foot
Calcaneus	Heel bone
Talus	Uppermost of tarsals; articulates with tibia and fibula; boxed in medial and lateral malleoli
Longitudinal arches	Tarsals and metatarsals so arranged as to form arch from front to back of foot
Medial	Formed by calcaneus, talus, navicular, cuneiforms, and three medial metatarsals
Lateral	Formed by calcaneus, cuboid, and two lateral metatarsals
Transverse (or metatarsal) arch	Metatarsals and distal row of tarsals (cuneiforms and cuboid) so articulated as to form arch across foot; bones kept in two arched positions by means of powerful ligaments in sole of foot and by muscles and tendons
Metatarsals	Long bones of feet
Phalanges	Miniature long bones of toes; two in each great toe; three in other toes

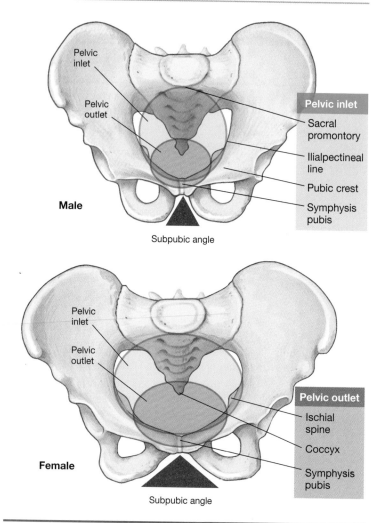

Figure 2-18 **Comparison of male and female bony pelvis.**

Table 2-11	Comparison of Male and Female Skeletons	
PORTION OF SKELETON	**MALE**	**FEMALE**
General form	Bones heavier and thicker; muscle attachment sites more massive; joint surfaces relatively large	Bones lighter and thinner; muscle attachment sites less distinct; joint surfaces relatively small

Table 2-11	Comparison of Male and Female Skeletons—cont'd	
PORTION OF SKELETON	**MALE**	**FEMALE**
Skull	Forehead shorter vertically; mandible and maxillae relatively larger; facial area more pronounced; processes more prominent	Forehead more elongated vertically; mandible and maxillae relatively smaller; facial area rounder, with less pronounced features; processes less pronounced
Pelvis		
Pelvic cavity	Narrower in all dimensions; deeper; pelvic outlet relatively small	Wider in all dimensions; shorter and roomier; pelvic outlet relatively large
Sacrum	Long, narrow, with smooth concavity (sacral curvature); sacral promontory more pronounced	Short, wide, flat concavity more pronounced in a posterior direction; sacral promontory less pronounced
Coccyx	Less movable	More movable and follows posterior direction of sacral curvature
Pubic arch	60- to 90-degree angle	90- to 120-degree angle
Symphysis pubis	Relatively deep	Relatively shallow
Ischial spine, ischial tuberosity, and anterior superior iliac spine	Turned more inward	Turned more outward and further apart
Greater sciatic notch	Narrow	Wide

Table 2-12	Primary Joint Classifications		
FUNCTIONAL NAME	**STRUCTURAL NAME**	**MOVEMENT PERMITTED**	**EXAMPLE**
Synarthroses	Fibrous	Immovable	Sutures of skull
Amphiarthroses	Cartilaginous	Slightly movable	Symphysis pubis
Diarthroses	Synovial	Freely movable	Shoulder joint

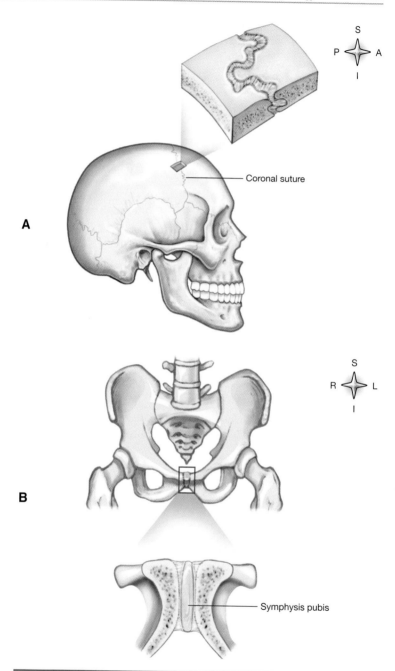

Figure 2-19 **Joints of the skeleton. A,** Example of a fibrous, synarthrotic joint. **B,** Example of a cartilaginous, amphiarthrotic joint.

Table 2-13	Classification of Fibrous and Cartilaginous Joints		
TYPES	**EXAMPLES**	**STRUCTURAL FEATURES**	**MOVEMENT**
Fibrous Joints			
Syndesmoses	Joints between distal ends of radius and ulna	Fibrous bands (ligaments) connect articulating bones	Slight
Sutures	Joints between skull bones	Teethlike projections of articulating bones interlock with thin layer of fibrous tissue connecting them	None
Gomphoses	Joints between roots of teeth and jaw bones	Fibrous tissue connects roots of teeth to alveolar processes	None
Cartilaginous Joints			
Synchondroses	Costal cartilage attachments of first rib to sternum; epiphyseal plate between diaphysis and epiphysis of growing long bone	Hyaline cartilage connects articulating bones	Slight
Symphyses	Symphysis pubis; joints between bodies of vertebrae	Fibrocartilage between articulating bones	Slight

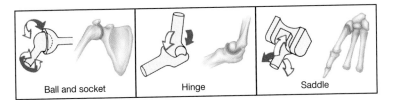

Ball and socket   Hinge   Saddle

Figure 2-20 Types of synovial, diarthrotic joints. Notice that the shapes of the articulating bones dictate the type of movement that is permitted at each joint.

Continued

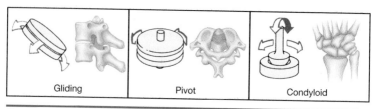

| Gliding | Pivot | Condyloid |

Figure 2-20—cont'd Types of synovial, diarthrotic joints. Notice that the shapes of the articulating bones dictate the type of movement that is permitted at each joint.

Table 2-14   Classification of Synovial Joints

TYPES	EXAMPLES	TYPE	MOVEMENT
Uniaxial			Around one axis; in one place
Hinge	Elbow joint	Spool-shaped process fits into concave socket	Flexion and extension only
Pivot	Joint between first and second cervical vertebrae	Arch-shaped process fits around peg-like process	Rotation
Biaxial			Around two axes, perpendicular to each other; in two planes
Saddle	Thumb joint between first metacarpal and carpal bone	Saddle-shaped bone fits into socket that is concave-convex-concave	Flexion, extension in one plane; abduction, adduction in other plane; opposing thumb to finger
Condyloid (ellipsoidal)	Joint between radius and carpal bones	Oval condyle fits into elliptic socket	Flexion, extension in one plane; abduction, adduction in other plane
Multiaxial			Around many axes
Ball and socket	Shoulder joint and hip	Ball-shaped process fits into concave socket	Widest range of movements; flexion, extension, abduction, adduction, rotation, circumduction

Table 2-14 — Classification of Synovial Joints—cont'd

TYPES	EXAMPLES	TYPE	MOVEMENT
Gliding	Joints between articular facets of adjacent vertebrae; joints between carpal and tarsal bones	Relatively flat articulating surfaces	Gliding movements without any angular or circular movements

Field Notes

Uncle Red, Freckles, and Muscles

I always loved holiday gatherings with my mom's extended family. I often saw relatives, relatives of relatives, and friends of relatives that I didn't otherwise get to visit. One of those folks was Uncle Red. That wasn't his real name—I still don't know his real name. They called him Red because he had brilliant red hair. It's what you noticed about him first. Whenever he came to a holiday party, he always brought his dog Freckles. Freckles was called that because he was a spaniel with lots of red dots on his white fur—making him look freckled.

The problem for me was that when they arrived everyone would call out, "Red and Freckles are here!" In would strut the happy dog, followed by his master; I always thought that the dog was "Red"— he WAS red in parts—and the man was "Freckles" because he did indeed have prominent red freckles on his face. I'm still not sure I have it right, but my mom insists that the man was Red and the dog was Freckles.

My point is that even though this one case confused me (and still does), most of the time such names are very helpful. We often use one or two physical features to name a person, an animal, or a building. We also use a similar system in naming muscles.

When you look at muscle names, you'll notice that they work like the nicknames we give people. Just as names like Big Al, Uncle Red, or Pastor Eddie tell you something about the way these people look or what they do, muscle names provide similar information. However, because muscle names are Latin in origin, you'll need to know that, for example, *maximus* means *big* and *minimus* means *small* and *adductor* means that *it pulls toward the midline of the body*.

Continued on page 140

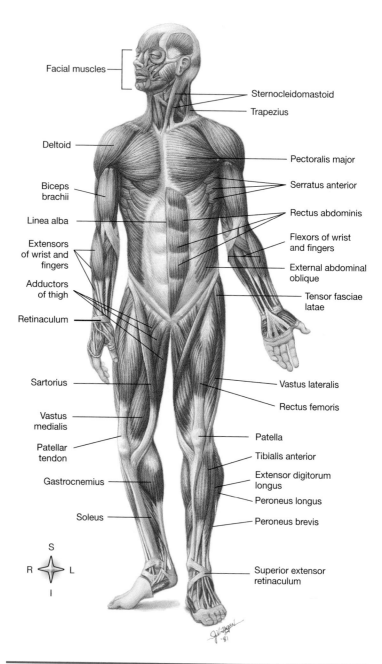

Facial muscles

Sternocleidomastoid

Trapezius

Deltoid

Pectoralis major

Biceps brachii

Serratus anterior

Linea alba

Rectus abdominis

Extensors of wrist and fingers

Flexors of wrist and fingers

Adductors of thigh

External abdominal oblique

Retinaculum

Tensor fasciae latae

Sartorius

Vastus lateralis

Rectus femoris

Vastus medialis

Patella

Patellar tendon

Tibialis anterior

Gastrocnemius

Extensor digitorum longus

Peroneus longus

Soleus

Peroneus brevis

S

R L

I

Superior extensor retinaculum

Figure 2-21 General overview of the body musculature. Anterior view.

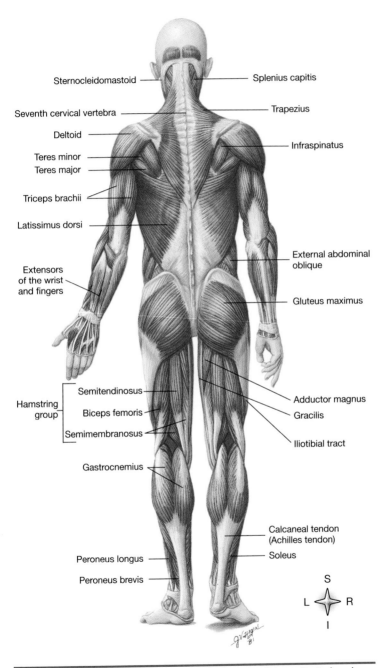

Figure 2-22 General overview of the body musculature. Posterior view.

Field Notes—cont'd

Uncle Red, Freckles, and Muscles—cont'd

The next several tables list some of these designations. If you take the time to become familiar with them, you'll find the muscle names easy to remember (because they'll make sense to you). You'll also find that it will be easy to find them in the body or figure out their actions.

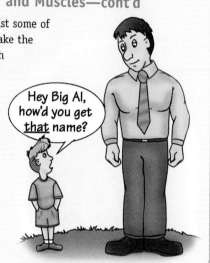

Hey Big Al, how'd you get _that_ name?

Table 2-15   Selected Muscles Grouped According to Function

PART MOVED	EXAMPLE OF FLEXOR	EXAMPLE OF EXTENSOR	EXAMPLE OF ABDUCTOR	EXAMPLE OF ADDUCTOR
Head	Sternocleido-mastoid	Semispinalis capitis		
Upper arm	Pectoralis major	Trapezius, latissimus dorsi	Deltoid	Pectoralis major with latissimus dorsi
Forearm	With forearm supinated: biceps brachii; with forearm pronated: brachialis; with semisupination or semiprona-tion: brachio-radialis	Triceps brachii		

Table 2-15	Selected Muscles Grouped According to Function—cont'd			
PART MOVED	EXAMPLE OF FLEXOR	EXAMPLE OF EXTENSOR	EXAMPLE OF ABDUCTOR	EXAMPLE OF ADDUCTOR
Hand	Flexor carpi radialis and ulnaris; palmaris longus	Extensor carpi radialis, longus, and brevis; extensor carpi ulnaris	Flexor carpi radialis	Flexor carpi ulnaris
Thigh	Iliopsoas, rectus femoris (of quadriceps femoris group)	Gluteus maximus	Gluteus medius and gluteus minimus	Adductor group
Leg	Hamstrings	Quadriceps femoris group		
Foot	Tibialis anterior	Gastrocnemius, soleus	Evertors, peroneus longus, peroneus brevis	Invertor, tibialis anterior
Trunk	Iliopsoas, rectus abdominis	Erector spinae		

Table 2-16	Selected Muscles Grouped According to Shape	
NAME	MEANING	EXAMPLE
Deltoid	Triangular	Deltoid
Gracilis	Slender	Gracilis
Trapezius	Trapezoid	Trapezius
Serratus	Notched	Serratus anterior
Teres	Round	Pronator teres
Rhomboid	Rhomboidal	Rhomboid major
Orbicularis	Round or circular	Orbicularis oris
Pectinate	Comblike	Pectineus
Piriformis	Wedge-shaped	Piriformis
Platys	Flat	Platysma
Quadratus	Square	Quadratus femoris
Lumbrical	Wormlike	Lumbricals

Table 2-17 Selected Muscles Grouped According to Number of Heads and Direction of Fibers

NAME	MEANING	EXAMPLE
Number of Heads		
Biceps	Two heads	Biceps brachii
Triceps	Three heads	Triceps brachii
Quadriceps	Four heads	Quadriceps
Digastric	Two bellies	Digastric
Direction of Fibers		
Oblique	Diagonal	External oblique rectus
Rectus	Straight	Rectus abdominis
Transverse	Transverse	Transversus abdominis
Circular	Around	Orbicularis oris
Spiral	Oblique	Supinator

Table 2-19 Muscles of Facial Expression and of Mastication

MUSCLE	ORIGIN	INSERTION
Muscles of Facial Expression		
Occipitofrontalis (epicranius)	Occipital bone	Tissues of eyebrows
Corrugator supercilii	Frontal bone (superciliary ridge)	Skin of eyebrow
Orbicularis oculi	Encircles eyelid	
Zygomaticus major	Zygomatic bone	Angle of mouth
Orbicularis oris	Encircles mouth	
Buccinator	Maxillae	Skin of sides of mouth
Muscles of Mastication		
Masseter	Zygomatic arch	Mandible (external surface)
Temporalis	Temporal bone	Mandible
Pterygoids (lateral and medial)	Undersurface of skull	Mandible (medial surface)

Table 2-18	Selected Muscles Grouped According to Size	
NAME	**MEANING**	**EXAMPLE**
Major	Large	Pectoralis major
Maximus	Largest	Gluteus maximus
Minor	Small	Pectoralis minor
Minimus	Smallest	Gluteus minimus
Longus	Long	Adductor longus
Brevis	Short	Extensor pollicis brevis
Latissimus	Very wide	Latissimus dorsi
Longissimus	Very long	Longissimus
Magnus	Very large	Adductor magnus
Vastus	Vast or huge	Vastus medialis

FUNCTION	**NERVE SUPPLY**
Raises eyebrows; wrinkles forehead horizontally	Cranial nerve VII
Wrinkles forehead vertically	Cranial nerve VII
Closes eye	Cranial nerve VII
Laughing (elevates angle of mouth)	Cranial nerve VII
Draws lips together	Cranial nerve VII
Permits smiling; blowing, as in playing a trumpet	Cranial nerve VII
Closes jaw	Cranial nerve V
Closes jaw	Cranial nerve V
Grates teeth	Cranial nerve V

Table 2-20　Muscles That Move the Head

MUSCLE	ORIGIN	INSERTION
Sternocleidomastoid	Sternum	Temporal bone (mastoid process)
	Clavicle	
Semispinalis capitis	Vertebrae (transverse processes of upper six thoracic; articular processes of lower four cervical)	Occipital bone (between superior and inferior nuchal lines)
Splenius capitis	Ligamentum nuchae	Temporal bone (mastoid process)
	Vertebrae (spinous processes of upper three or four thoracic)	Occipital bone
Longissimus capitis	Vertebrae (transverse processes of upper six thoracic; articular processes of lower four cervical)	Temporal bone (mastoid process)

Table 2-21　Muscles of the Thorax

MUSCLE	ORIGIN	INSERTION
External intercostals	Rib (lower border; forward fibers)	Rib (upper border of rib below origin)
Internal intercostals	Rib (inner surface, lower border; backward fibers)	Rib (upper border of rib below origin)
Diaphragm	Lower circumference of thorax (of rib cage)	Central tendon of diaphragm

FUNCTION	NERVE SUPPLY
Flexes head (prayer muscle)	Accessory nerve
One muscle alone, rotates head toward opposite side; spasm of this muscle alone or associated with trapezius called *torticollis* or *wryneck*	
Extends head; bends it laterally	First five cervical nerves
Extends head	Second, third, and fourth cervical nerves
Bends and rotates head toward same side as contracting muscle	
Extends head	Multiple innervation
Bends and rotates head toward contracting side	

FUNCTION	NERVE SUPPLY
Elevate ribs	Intercostal nerves
Depress ribs	Intercostal nerves
Enlarges thorax, causing inspiration	Phrenic nerves

Table 2-22   Muscles of the Abdominal Wall

MUSCLE	ORIGIN	INSERTION
External oblique	Ribs (lower eight)	Pelvis (iliac crest and pubis by way of inguinal ligament)
		Linea alba by way of an aponeurosis
Internal oblique	Pelvis (iliac crest and inguinal ligament)	Ribs (lower three)
	Lumbodorsal fascia	Linea alba
Transversus abdominis	Ribs (lower six)	Pubic bone
	Pelvis (iliac crest, inguinal ligament)	Linea alba
	Lumbodorsal fascia	Ribs (costal cartilage of fifth, sixth, and seventh ribs)
Rectus abdominis	Pelvis (pubic bone and symphysis pubis)	Sternum (xiphoid process)
Quadratus lumborum	Iliolumbar ligament; iliac crest	Last rib; transverse process of vertebrae (L1-L4)

FUNCTION	NERVE SUPPLY
Compresses abdomen	Lower seven intercostal nerves and iliohypogastric nerves
Rotates trunk laterally	
Important postural function of all abdominal muscles is to pull front of pelvis upward, thereby flattening lumbar curve of spine; when these muscles lose their tone, common figure faults of protruding abdomen and lordosis develop	
Same as external oblique	Last three intercostal nerves; iliohypogastric and ilioinguinal nerves
Same as external oblique	Last five intercostal nerves; iliohypogastric and ilioinguinal nerves
Same as external oblique; because abdominal muscles compress abdominal cavity, they aid in straining, defecation, forced expiration, and childbirth; abdominal muscles are antagonists of diaphragm, relaxing as it contracts and vice versa	Last six intercostal nerves
Flexes trunk	
Flexes vertebral column laterally; depresses last rib	Lumbar

Table 2-23   Muscles of the Back

MUSCLE	ORIGIN	INSERTION
Erector Spinae Group		
Iliocostalis group	Various regions of the pelvis and ribs	Ribs and vertebra (superior to origin)
Longissimus group	Cervical and thoracic vertebrae, ribs	Mastoid process, upper cervical vertebrae, or upper lumbar vertebrae
Spinalis group	Lower cervical or lower thoracic/upper lumbar vertebrae	Upper cervical or middle/upper thoracic vertebrae (superior to origin)
Transversospinalis Group		
Semispinalis group	Transverse processes of vertebrae (T2-T11)	Spinous processes of vertebrae (C2-T4)
Multifidus group	Transverse processes of vertebrae; sacrum and ilium	Spinous processes of (next superior) vertebrae
Rotatores group	Transverse processes of vertebrae	Spinous processes of (next superior) vertebrae
Splenius	Spinous processes of vertebrae (C7-T1 or T3-T6)	Lateral occipital/mastoid or transverse processes of vertebrae (C1-C4)
Interspinales group	Spinous processes of vertebrae	Spinous processes (of next superior vertebrae)

Table 2-24   Muscles of the Pelvic Floor

MUSCLE	ORIGIN	INSERTION
Levator ani	Pubis and spine of ischium	Coccyx
Ischiocavernosus	Ischium	Penis or clitoris
Bulbospongiosus	*In males:* Bulb of penis *In females:* Perineum	Perineum and bulb of penis Base of clitoris
Deep transverse perinea	Ischium	Central tendon (median raphe)
Sphincter urethrae	Pubic ramus	Central tendon (median raphe)
Sphincter ani externus	Coccyx	Central tendon (median raphe)

FUNCTION	NERVE SUPPLY
Extends, laterally flexes vertebral column	Spinal, thoracic, or lumbar nerves
Extends head, neck, or vertebral column	Cervical or thoracic and lumbar nerves
Extends neck or vertebral column	Cervical or thoracic nerves
Extends neck or vertebral column	Cervical or thoracic nerves
Extends, rotates vertebral column	Spinal nerves
Extends, rotates vertebral column	Spinal nerves
Rotates, extends neck and flexes neck laterally	Cervical nerves
Extends back and neck	Spinal nerves

FUNCTION	NERVE SUPPLY
Together with coccygeus muscles form floor of pelvic cavity and support pelvic organs	Pudendal nerve
Compress base of penis or clitoris	Perineal nerve
Constricts urethra and erects penis Erects clitoris	Pudendal nerve Pudendal nerve
Support pelvic floor	Pudendal nerve
Constrict urethra	Pudendal nerve
Close anal canal	Pudendal and S4

Table 2-25	Muscles Acting on the Shoulder Girdle	
MUSCLE	**ORIGIN**	**INSERTION**
Trapezius	Occipital bone (protuberance)	Clavicle
	Vertebrae (cervical and thoracic)	Scapula (spine and acromion)
Pectoralis minor	Ribs (second to fifth)	Scapula (coracoid)
Serratus anterior	Ribs (upper eight or nine)	Scapula (anterior surface, vertebral border)
Levator scapulae	C1-C4 (transverse processes)	Scapula (superior angle)
Rhomboid	*Major:* T1-T4 *Minor:* C6-C7	Scapula (medial border) Scapula (medial border)

Table 2-26	Muscles That Move the Upper Arm	
MUSCLE	**ORIGIN**	**INSERTION**
Axial*		
Pectoralis major	Clavicle (medial half)	Humerus (greater tubercle)
	Sternum	
	Costal cartilages of true ribs	
Latissimus dorsi	Vertebrae (spines of lower thoracic, lumbar, and sacral)	Humerus (intertubercular groove)
	Ilium (crest)	
	Lumbodorsal fascia	
Scapular*		
Deltoid	Clavicle	Humerus (lateral side about halfway down—deltoid tubercle)
	Scapula (spine and acromion)	
Coracobrachialis	Scapula (coracoid process)	Humerus (middle third, medial surface)

Axial muscles originate on the axial skeleton; *scapular* muscles originate on the scapula.

FUNCTION	NERVE SUPPLY
Raises or lowers shoulders and shrugs them	Spinal accessory; second, third, and fourth cervical nerves
Extends head when occiput acts as insertion	
Pulls shoulder down and forward	Medial and lateral anterior thoracic nerves
Pulls shoulder down and forward; abducts and rotates it upward	Long thoracic nerve
Elevates and retracts scapula and abducts neck	Dorsal scapular nerve
Retracts, rotates, fixes scapula	Dorsal scapular nerve
Retracts, rotates, elevates, and fixes scapula	Dorsal scapular nerve

FUNCTION	NERVE SUPPLY
Flexes upper arm	Medial and lateral anterior thoracic nerves
Adducts upper arm anteriorly; draws it across chest	
Extends upper arm; adducts upper arm posteriorly	Thoracodorsal nerve
Abducts upper arm	Axillary nerve
Assists in flexion and extension of upper arm	
Adduction; assists in flexion and medial rotation of arm	Musculocutaneous nerve

Continued

Table 2-26   Muscles That Move the Upper Arm—cont'd

MUSCLE	ORIGIN	INSERTION
Supraspinatus[†]	Scapula (supraspinous fossa)	Humerus (greater tubercle)
Teres minor[†]	Scapula (axillary border)	Humerus (greater tubercle)
Teres major	Scapula (lower part, axillary border)	Humerus (upper part, anterior surface)
Infraspinatus[†]	Scapula (infraspinatus border)	Humerus (greater tubercle)
Subscapularis[†]	Scapula (subscapular fossa)	Humerus (lesser tubercle)

[†]Muscles of the rotator cuff.

Table 2-27   Muscles That Move the Forearm

MUSCLE	ORIGIN	INSERTION
Flexors		
Biceps brachii	Scapula (supraglenoid tuberosity)	Radius (tubercle at proximal end)
	Scapula (coracoid)	
Brachialis	Humerus (distal half, anterior surface)	Ulna (front of coronoid process)
Brachioradialis	Humerus (above lateral epicondyle)	Radius (styloid process)
Extensor		
Triceps brachii	Scapula (infraglenoid tuberosity)	Ulna (olecranon process)
	Humerus (posterior surface—lateral head above radial groove; medial head, below)	
Pronators		
Pronator teres	Humerus (medial epicondyle)	Radius (middle third of lateral surface)

FUNCTION	NERVE SUPPLY
Assists in abducting arm	Suprascapular nerve
Rotates arm outward	Axillary nerve
Assists in extension, adduction, and medial rotation of arm	Lower subscapular nerve
Rotates arm outward	Suprascapular nerve
Medial rotation	Suprascapular nerve

FUNCTION	NERVE SUPPLY
Flexes supinated forearm	Musculocutaneous nerve
Supinates forearm and hand	
Flexes pronated forearm	Musculocutaneous nerve
Flexes semipronated or semi-supinated forearm; supinates forearm and hand	Radial nerve
Extends lower arm	Radial nerve
Pronates and flexes forearm	Median nerve

Continued

Table 2-27   Muscles That Move the Forearm—cont'd

MUSCLE	ORIGIN	INSERTION
	Ulna (coronoid process)	
Pronator quadratus	Ulna (distal fourth, anterior surface)	Radius (distal fourth, anterior surface)
Supinator		
Supinator	Humerus (lateral epicondyle)	Radius (proximal third)
	Ulna (proximal fifth)	

Table 2-28   Muscles That Move the Wrist, Hand, and Fingers

MUSCLE	ORIGIN	INSERTION
Extrinsic		
Flexor carpi radialis	Humerus (medial epicondyle)	Second metacarpal (base of)
Palmaris longus	Humerus (medial epicondyle)	Fascia of palm
Flexor carpi ulnaris	Humerus (medial epicondyle)	Pisiform bone
	Ulna (proximal two thirds)	Third, fourth, and fifth metacarpals
Extensor carpi radialis longus	Humerus (ridge above lateral epicondyle)	Second metacarpal (base of)
Extensor carpi radialis brevis	Humerus (lateral epicondyle)	Second, third metacarpals (bases of)
Extensor carpi ulnaris	Humerus (lateral epicondyle)	Fifth metacarpal (base of)
	Ulna (proximal three fourths)	Adducts hand (moves toward little finger side when hand supinated)
Flexor digitorum profundus	Ulna (anterior surface)	Distal phalanges (fingers two to five)
Flexor digitorum superficialis	Humerus (medial epicondyle)	Tendons of fingers

FUNCTION	NERVE SUPPLY
Pronates forearm	Median nerve
Supinates forearm	Radial nerve

FUNCTION	NERVE SUPPLY
Flexes hand; flexes forearm	Median nerve
Flexes hand	Median nerve
Flexes hand	Ulnar nerve
Adducts hand	
Extends hand; abducts hand (moves toward thumb side when hand supinated)	Radial nerve
Extends hand	Radial nerve
Extends hand	Radial nerve
Flexes distal interphalangeal joints	Median and ulnar nerves
Flexes fingers	Median nerve

Continued

Table 2-28 Muscles That Move the Wrist, Hand, and Fingers—cont

MUSCLE	ORIGIN	INSERTION
	Radius	
	Ulna (coronoid process)	
Extensor digitorum	Humerus (lateral epicondyle)	Phalanges (fingers two to five)
Intrinsic		
Opponens pollicis	Trapezium	Thumb metacarpal
Abductor pollicis brevis	Trapezium	Proximal phalanx of thumb
Adductor pollicis	Second and third metacarpals	Proximal phalanx of thumb
	Trapezoid	
	Capitate	
Flexor pollicis brevis	Flexor retinaculum	Proximal phalanx of thumb
Abductor digiti minimi	Pisiform	Proximal phalanx of fifth finger
Flexor digiti minimi brevis	Hamate	Proximal and middle phalanx of fifth finger
Opponens digiti minimi	Hamate	Fifth metacarpal
	Flexor retinaculum	
Interosseous (palmar and dorsal)	Metacarpals	Proximal phalanges
Lumbricals	Tendons of flexor digitorum profundus	Phalanges (two to five)

FUNCTION	NERVE SUPPLY
Extends fingers	Radial nerve
Opposes thumb to fingers	Median nerve
Abducts thumb	Median nerve
Adducts thumb	Ulnar nerve
Flexes thumb	Median and ulnar nerves
Abducts fifth finger	Ulnar nerve
Flexes fifth finger	
Flexes fifth finger	Ulnar nerve
Opposes fifth finger slightly	Ulnar nerve
Adducts second, fourth, fifth fingers (palmar)	Ulnar nerve
Abducts second, third, fourth fingers (dorsal)	
Flexes proximal phalanges (two to five)	Median nerve (phalanges two and three)
Extends middle and distal phalanges (two to five)	Ulnar nerve (phalanges four and five)

Table 2-29	Muscles That Move the Thigh	
MUSCLE	**ORIGIN**	**INSERTION**
Iliopsoas (iliacus, psoas major, psoas minor)	Ilium (iliac fossa)	Femur (lesser trochanter)
	Vertebrae (bodies of twelfth thoracic to fifth lumbar)	
Rectus femoris	Ilium (anterior, inferior spine)	Tibia (by way of patellar tendon)
Gluteal Group		
Maximus	Ilium (crest and posterior surface)	Femur (gluteal tuberosity)
	Sacrum and coccyx (posterior surface); sacrotuberous ligament	Iliotibial tract
Medius	Ilium (lateral surface)	Femur (greater trochanter)
Minimus	Ilium (lateral surface)	Femur (greater trochanter)
Tensor fasciae latae	Ilium (anterior part of crest)	Tibia (by way of iliotibial tract)
Adductor Group		
Brevis	Pubic bone	Femur (linea aspera)
Longus	Pubic bone	Femur (linea aspera)
Magnus	Pubic bone	Femur (linea aspera)
Gracilis	Pubic bone (just below symphysis)	Tibia (medial surface behind sartorius)

FUNCTION	NERVE SUPPLY
Flexes thigh	Femoral and second to fourth lumbar nerves
Flexes trunk (when femur acts as origin)	
Flexes thigh	Femoral nerve
Extends lower leg	
Extends thigh—rotates outward	Inferior gluteal nerve
Abducts thigh—rotates outward; stabilizes pelvis on femur	Superior gluteal nerve
Abducts thigh; stabilizes pelvis on femur; rotates thigh medially	Superior gluteal nerve
Abducts thigh; tightens iliotibial tract	Superior gluteal nerve
Adducts thigh	Obturator nerve
Adducts thigh	Obturator nerve
Adducts thigh	Obturator nerve
Adducts thigh and flexes and adducts leg	Obturator nerve

Table 2-30	Muscles That Move the Lower Leg	
MUSCLE	**ORIGIN**	**INSERTION**
Quadriceps Femoris Group		
Rectus femoris	Ilium (anterior inferior spine)	Tibia (by way of patellar tendon)
Vastus lateralis	Femur (linea aspera)	Tibia (by way of patellar tendon)
Vastus medialis	Femur	Tibia (by way of patellar tendon)
Vastus intermedius	Femur (anterior surface)	Tibia (by way of patellar tendon)
Sartorius	Coxal (anterior, superior iliac spines)	Tibia (medial surface of upper end of shaft)
Hamstring Group		
Biceps femoris	Ischium (tuberosity)	Fibula (head of)
	Femur (linea aspera)	Tibia (lateral condyle)
Semitendinosus	Ischium (tuberosity)	Tibia (proximal end, medial surface)
Semimembranosus	Ischium (tuberosity)	Tibia (medial condyle)

Table 2-31	Muscles That Move the Foot	
MUSCLE	**ORIGIN**	**INSERTION**
Extrinsic		
Tibialis anterior	Tibia (lateral condyle of upper body)	Tarsal (first cuneiform)
		Metatarsal (base of first)
Gastrocnemius	Femur (condyles)	Tarsal (calcaneus by way of Achilles tendon)
Soleus	Tibia (underneath gastrocnemius)	Tarsal (calcaneus by way of Achilles tendon)
	Fibula	
Peroneus longus	Tibia (lateral condyle)	First cuneiform
	Fibula (head and shaft)	Base of first metatarsal
Peroneus brevis	Fibula (lower two thirds of lateral surface of shaft)	Fifth metatarsal (tubercle, dorsal surface)

FUNCTION	NERVE SUPPLY
Flexes thigh; extends leg	Femoral nerve
Extends leg	Femoral nerve
Extends leg	Femoral nerve
Extends leg	Femoral nerve
Adducts and flexes leg; permits crossing of legs tailor fashion	Femoral nerve
Extends thigh	Hamstring nerve (branch of sciatic nerve)
	Hamstring nerve
Extends thigh	Hamstring nerve
Extends thigh	Hamstring nerve

FUNCTION	NERVE SUPPLY
Flexes foot	Common and deep peroneal nerves
Inverts foot	
Extends foot; flexes lower leg	Tibial nerve (branch of sciatic nerve)
Extends foot (plantar flexion)	Tibial nerve
Extends foot (plantar flexion)	Common peroneal nerve
Everts foot	
Everts foot; flexes foot	Superficial peroneal nerve

Continued

Table 2-31   Muscles That Move the Foot—cont'd

MUSCLE	ORIGIN	INSERTION
Peroneus tertius	Fibula (distal third)	Fourth and fifth metatarsals (bases of)
Extensor digitorum longus	Tibia (lateral condyle)	Second and third phalanges (four lateral toes)
	Fibula (anterior surface)	
Intrinsic		
Lumbricals	Tendons of flexor digitorum longus	Phalanges (two to five)
Flexor digiti minimi brevis	Fifth metatarsal	Proximal phalanx of fifth toe
Flexor hallucis brevis	Cuboid	Proximal phalanx of first (great) toe
	Medial and lateral cuneiform	
Flexor digitorum brevis	Calcaneus	Middle phalanges of toes (two to five)
	Plantar fascia	
Abductor digiti minimi	Calcaneus	Proximal phalanx of fifth (small) toe
Abductor hallucis	Calcaneus	First (great) toe

FUNCTION	NERVE SUPPLY
Flexes foot; everts foot	Deep peroneal nerve
Dorsiflexion of foot; extension of toes	Deep peroneal nerve
Flex proximal phalanges; extend middle and distal phalanges	Lateral and medial plantar nerve
Flexes fifth (small) toe	Lateral plantar nerve
Flexes first (great) toe	Medial and lateral plantar nerve
Flexes toes two through five	Medial plantar nerve
Abducts fifth (small) toe; flexes fifth toe	Lateral plantar nerve
Abducts first (great) toe	Medial plantar nerve

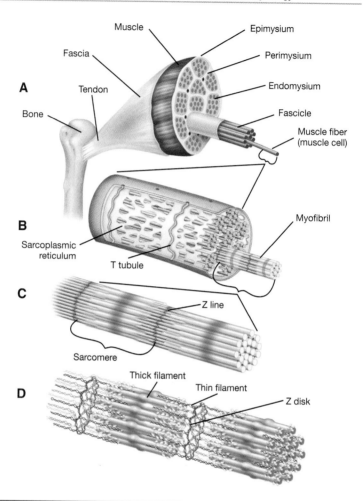

Figure 2-23 Structure of skeletal muscle. A, Skeletal muscle organ, composed of bundles of contractile muscle fibers held together by connective tissue. **B,** Greater magnification of single fiber showing smaller fibers—myofibrils—in the sarcoplasm. Note sarcoplasmic reticulum and T tubules forming a three-part structure called a triad. **C,** Myofibril magnified further to show sarcomere between successive Z lines. Cross striae are visible. **D,** Molecular structure of myofibril showing thick myofilaments and thin myofilaments. Z line is also called Z disk.

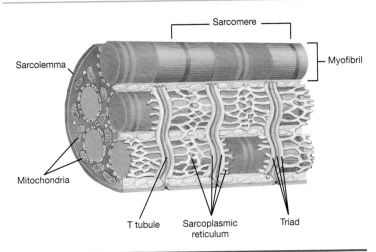

Figure 2-24 Unique features of the skeletal muscle fiber. Notice especially the T tubules, which are extensions of the plasma membrane, or sarcolemma, and the sarcoplasmic reticulum (SR), a type of smooth endoplasmic reticulum that forms networks of tubular canals and sacs containing stored calcium ions. A triad is a triplet of adjacent tubules: a terminal *(end)* sac of the SR, a T tubule, and another terminal sac of the SR. Cylindric sections of the cytoskeleton called myofibrils are made up of thick and thin myofilaments *(see Figure 2-23)*. Numerous mitochondria in the muscle fiber *(muscle cell)* transfer energy to adenosine triphosphate (ATP) to supply the high energy consumption of muscular contraction.

Box 2-1

Major Events of Skeletal Muscle Contraction and Relaxation

Excitation and Contraction

1. A nerve impulse reaches the end of a motor neuron, triggering the release of the neurotransmitter acetylcholine.
2. Acetylcholine diffuses rapidly across the gap of the neuromuscular junction and binds to acetylcholine receptors on the motor endplate of the muscle fiber.
3. Stimulation of acetylcholine receptors initiates impulses that travel along the sarcolemma, through the T tubules, to the sacs of the sarcoplasmic reticulum (SR).
4. Calcium (Ca) is released from the SR into the sarcoplasm, where it binds to troponin molecules in the thin myofilaments.
5. Tropomyosin molecules in the thin myofilaments shift, exposing actin's active sites.

Continued

Box 2-1

Major Events of Skeletal Muscle Contraction and Relaxation—cont'd

6. Energized myosin cross-bridges of the thick myofilaments bind to actin and use their energy to pull the thin myofilaments toward the center of each sarcomere. This cycle repeats itself many times per second, as long as adenosine triphosphate (ATP) is available.
7. As the filaments slide past the thick myofilaments, the entire muscle fiber shortens.

Relaxation

1. After the impulse is over, the SR begins actively pumping Ca^- back into its sacs.
2. As Ca^- is stripped from troponin molecules in the thin myofilaments, tropomyosin returns to its position, blocking actin's active sites.
3. Myosin cross-bridges are prevented from binding to actin and thus can no longer sustain the contraction.
4. Because the thick and thin myofilaments are no longer connected, the muscle fiber may return to its longer, resting length.

Field Notes

The Muscle Love Story

The molecular processes of the muscle fiber that produce "contraction" of a muscle are still not completely understood. Therefore it's no wonder that beginning students sometimes have a hard time understanding it. Analogies are a good way to learn physiologic processes. Here is my favorite analogy for muscle contraction, in the form of a love story:

The story begins in the land of the muscle fiber, where several interesting characters live. Myosin is in love with the girl next door, Actin. The problem is that some of the villagers want to keep Myosin and Actin apart (young lovers are never a likely match, according to others, are they?). A group of women, each called Troponin, constantly try to keep Myosin from getting to his true love (Actin) by holding up poles made of tropomyosin. These tropomyosin poles could be easily knocked out of the way by the brave and strong Myosin, but all those Troponin girls are very strong, too, and they keep the tropomyosin in its blocking position.

Every good love story needs tension like that—something keeping the lovers apart. In addition, there is a good subplot—the Troponin

Field Notes—cont'd

girls are in love, too. They each pine away for their true love—a Calcium. The problem for them is worse than for Actin and Myosin. All the Calciums are under guard in the SR (sarcoplasmic reticulum). The SR happens to be a sort of prison yard on the banks of the rivers, which the villagers call T tubules. Given their situation, it's very unlikely that any of the Troponins will ever be visited by a distant Calcium imprisoned in the SR. Poor things.

However, one day an odd thing happens—as it always does in these stories. A stranger (of course) called Acetylcholine is sent by the governing nervous system. Acetylcholine, or Ach to his friends, hits the sarcolemma, which is the wall around the village. That launches a traveling voltage fluctuation. You and I would call it an action potential, but the villagers think of it as a lightning strike.

Well, that voltage travels right along the sarcolemma and when it gets to each of the T tubules, it travels right down the T tubules and thus criss-crosses the village. As it travels down each T tubule, the voltage zaps the SR—which sure does startle the guards. The guards are so stunned that they let many of the Calciums escape and run all over the village. Oh my!

The Troponins, of course, can hardly believe it! They dreamt last night that they were surrounded by Calciums—and lo, it has happened! The Calciums and the Troponins embrace and in the heat of

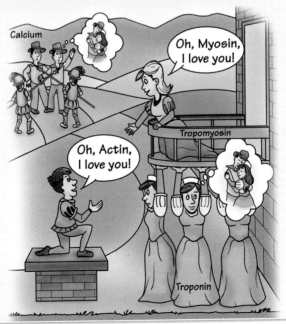

Field Notes—cont'd

passion twist around a little, completely forgetting about holding up the tropomyosin poles.

Well, that gives Myosin the chance he and Actin have been waiting for! He moves across the barrier and Myosin and Actin immediately start, well, getting passionate with each other. Myosin is very excited and just keeps Actin moving along. (I'd get into sliding filaments here, but it's a family book, OK?) You get the picture—we have contraction because Actin is being actively pulled along by Myosin, who is using a lot of energy.

In the meantime, back at the SR the guards have recovered and are now rounding up the Calciums and taking them back to the SR where they belong. As each Troponin tearfully bids her Calcium goodbye, she realizes that she was not paying attention to her job and gets back to it. So the next time Myosin is ready to cross over to Actin, he can't—he's again blocked by tropomyosin, which is being held in place by the Troponins.

Thus the little village returns to its relaxed state. If you can call it that—because all the old attractions are still there, and someday Ach will again ride to town and stir up an electrical storm.

Table 2-32 — Characteristics of Major Muscle Tissue Types

	SKELETAL	CARDIAC	SMOOTH
Principal location	Skeletal muscle organs	Wall of heart	Walls of many hollow organs
Principal functions	Movement of bones, heat production, posture	Pumping of blood	Movement in walls of hollow organs (peristalsis, mixing)
Type of control	Voluntary	Involuntary	Involuntary
Structural Features			
Striations	Present	Present	Absent
Nucleus	Many near sarcolemma	Single	Single; near center of cell
T tubules	Narrow; form triads with sarcoplasmic reticulum (SR)	Large diameter; form diads with SR, regulate calcium (Ca) entry into sarcoplasm	Absent

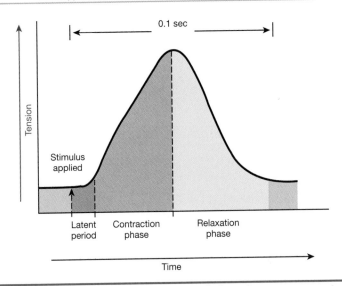

Figure 2-25 **The twitch contraction.** Three distinct phases are apparent: (1) the latent period, (2) the contraction phase, and (3) the relaxation phase.

Table 2-32	Characteristics of Major Muscle Tissue Types—cont'd		
	SKELETAL	**CARDIAC**	**SMOOTH**
Sarcoplasmic reticulum	Extensive; stores and releases Ca^{++}	Less extensive than in skeletal muscle	Very poorly developed
Cell junctions	No gap junctions	Intercalated disks	*Visceral:* Many gap junctions *Multiunit:* Few gap junctions
Contraction	Rapid twitch contractions of motor units usually consummate to produce sustained titanic contractions; must be stimulated by a neuron	Syncytium of fibers compress heart chambers in slow, separate contractions (does not exhibit tetanus or fatigue); exhibits autorhythmicity style	Visceral: Electrically coupled sheets of contract autorhythmically, producing peristalsis or mixing movements Multiunit: Individual fibers contract when stimulated by neuron

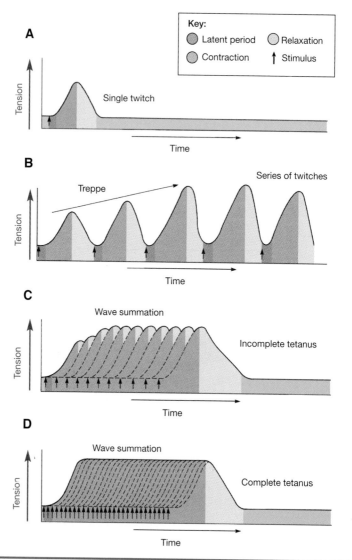

Figure 2-26 Myograms of various types of muscle contractions. A, A single-twitch contraction. **B,** The treppe phenomenon, or *staircase effect,* is a step-like increase in the force of contraction over the first few in a series of twitches. **C,** Incomplete tetanus occurs when a rapid succession of stimuli produces *twitches* that seem to add together (wave summation) to produce a rather sustained contraction. **D,** Complete tetanus is a smoother sustained contraction, produced by the summation of "twitches" that occur so close together that the muscle cannot relax at all.

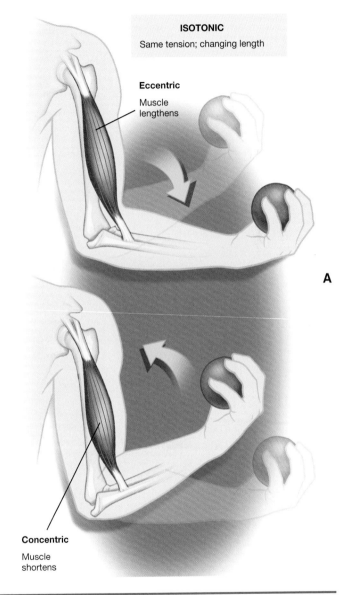

Figure 2-27 Isotonic and isometric contraction. A, In isotonic contraction, the muscle shortens, producing movement. Concentric contractions occur when the muscle shortens during the movement. Eccentric contractions occur when the contracting muscle lengthens.

Continued

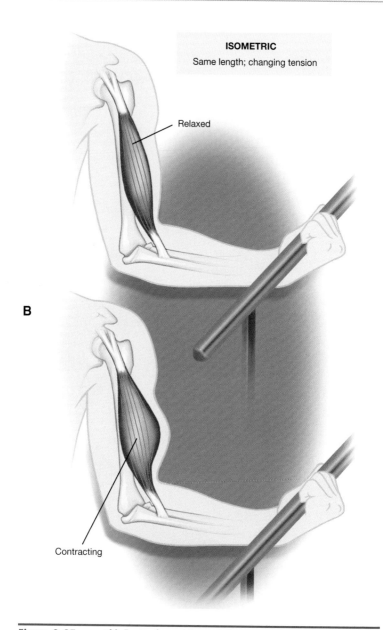

ISOMETRIC
Same length; changing tension

Relaxed

B

Contracting

Figure 2-27—cont'd **Isotonic and isometric contraction. B,** In isometric contraction the muscle pulls forcefully against a load but does not shorten.

Communication, Control, and Integration

3

TOPICS

Nervous system, endocrine system

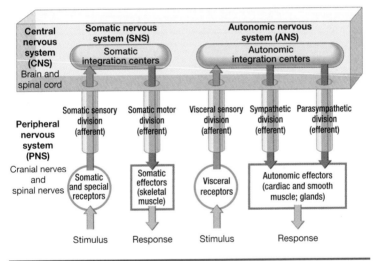

Figure 3-1 Organizational plan of the nervous system. The diagram
summarizes the scheme used by most neurobiologists in studying the
nervous system. Both the somatic nervous system (SNS) and the autonomic
nervous system (ANS) include components in the central nervous system
(CNS) and peripheral nervous system (PNS). Somatic sensory pathways
conduct information toward integrators in the CNS, and somatic motor
pathways conduct information toward somatic effectors. In the ANS, visceral
sensory pathways conduct information toward CNS integrators, whereas the
sympathetic and parasympathetic pathways conduct information toward
autonomic effectors.

Table 3-1	Types of Membrane Potentials		
MEMBRANE POTENTIAL	**POLARIZATION**	**TYPICAL VOLTAGE***	**SUMMATION**
Resting membrane potential	Polarized	−70 mV	Not applicable
Local potential	Depolarized (excitatory postsynaptic potential [EPSP])	Graded; varies higher than −70 mV	Yes
	Hyperpolarized (inhibitory postsynaptic potential [IPSP])	Graded; varies lower than −70 mV	Yes
Threshold potential	Depolarized	−59 mV	Yes
Action potential	Depolarized	+30 mV	No

*Example used in this chapter; actual values in body vary depending on many diverse factors.

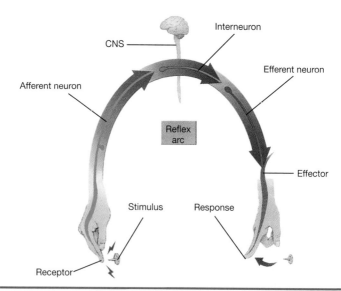

Figure 3-2 Reflex arc. Notice that the most basic route of signal conduction follows a pattern called the reflex arc. Neurons (nerve cells) can be classified functionally according to the direction in which they conduct impulses.

CONDUCTION	DESCRIPTION
Not applicable	Membrane voltage when the neuron is not excited and not conducting an impulse (RMP)
Decremental	Temporary fluctuation in a local region of the membrane in response to a sensory or nerve stimulus; may be an upward or downward fluctuation in voltage; loses amplitude as it spreads along membrane
Decremental	
Triggers action potential	Minimum local depolarization needed to trigger voltage-gated channels that produce the action potential
Nondecremental	Temporary maximum depolarization of membrane voltage that travels to end of axon without losing amplitude

Table 3-2   Steps of the Mechanism that Produces an Action Potential

STEP	DESCRIPTION
1	A stimulus triggers stimulus-gated sodium (Na^+) channels to open and allow inward Na^+ diffusion. This causes the membrane to depolarize.
2	As the threshold potential is reached, voltage-gated Na^+ channels open.
3	As more Na^+ enters the cell through voltage-gated Na^+ channels, the membrane depolarizes even further.
4	The magnitude of the action potential peaks (at $+30$ mV) when voltage-gated Na^+ channels close.
5	Repolarization begins when voltage-gated potassium (K^+) channels open, allowing outward diffusion of K^+.
6	After a brief period of hyperpolarization, the resting potential is restored by the sodium-potassium pump and the return of ion channels to their resting state.

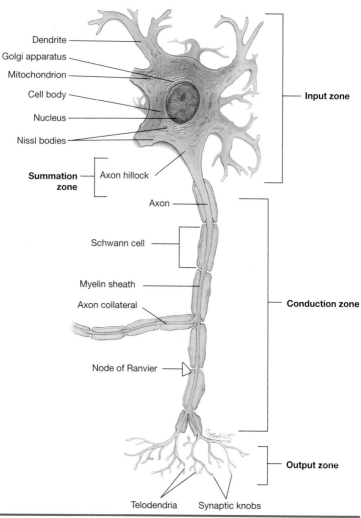

Dendrite

Golgi apparatus

Mitochondrion

Cell body

Nucleus

Nissl bodies

Summation zone

Axon hillock

Axon

Schwann cell

Myelin sheath

Axon collateral

Node of Ranvier

Telodendria   Synaptic knobs

Input zone

Conduction zone

Output zone

Figure 3-3 Structure of a typical neuron. Neurons consist of a cell body (perikaryon or soma) and at least two processes (nerve fibers): one axon and one or more dendrites. The dendrites and cell body act primarily as an input zone, receiving nerve stimulation and initiating nerve impulses in response. The axon extends from a tapered portion of the cell body called the axon hillock. The axon hillock acts as a summation zone by adding together all the nerve impulses arriving from the cell body and dendrites—and deciding whether to send the impulse any further. Axons conduct impulses away from the cell body and are the conduction zone. An axon often has one or more side branches (axon collaterals). The distal tips of axons form branches called *telodendria* that each terminate in a synaptic knob in the neuron. These end structures act as an output zone where vesicles of neurotransmitter are released.

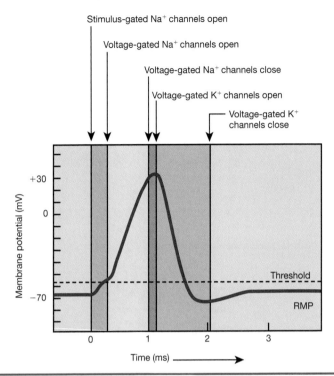

Stimulus-gated Na⁺ channels open

Voltage-gated Na⁺ channels open

Voltage-gated Na⁺ channels close

Voltage-gated K⁺ channels open

Voltage-gated K⁺ channels close

Figure 3-4 The action potential. Changes in membrane potential in a local area of a neuron's membrane result from changes in membrane permeability.

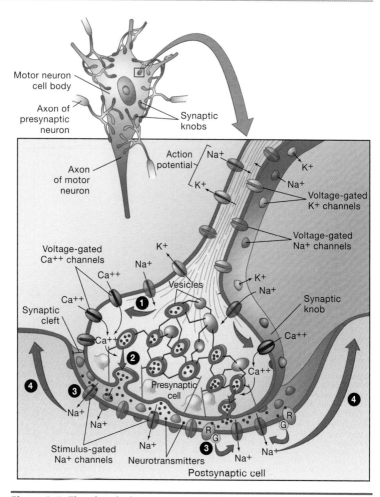

Figure 3-5 **The chemical synapse.** Detail of a synaptic knob, or axon terminal, of a presynaptic neuron, the plasma membrane of a postsynaptic neuron, and a synaptic cleft is shown. On the arrival of an action potential at a synaptic knob, voltage-gated calcium (Ca^{++}) channels open and allow extracellular Ca^{++} to diffuse into the presynaptic cell *(step 1)*. In *step 2*, the Ca^{++} triggers the rapid exocytosis of neurotransmitter molecules from vesicles in the knob. In *step 3*, the neurotransmitter diffuses into the synaptic cleft and binds to receptor molecules in the plasma membrane of the postsynaptic neuron. The postsynaptic receptors directly or indirectly trigger the opening of stimulus-gated ion channels, initiating a local potential in the postsynaptic neuron. In *step 4*, the local potential may move toward the axon, where an action potential may begin.

Field Notes

Sending Messages

As you can imagine, the ability to send messages is critical to the continued stable functioning of the human body. Nerve signals are sent by way of neurotransmitters; endocrine signals are sent by way of hormones; local signals are sent by way of paracrine or autocrine agents (local types of agents). The whole process of a cell's receiving and understanding any of these signals is called *signal transduction*.

Signal transduction is a really big deal. By that, I mean that if you really want to understand human physiology—and have any inkling of how most drugs and chemical therapies work—you have to know the basics of signal transduction. It's also a big deal because this is an area of intensely active and important scientific research.

Figures 3-6 and 3-7, which show different methods of signal transduction in postsynaptic cells, give us our first opportunity to learn the basics of this important concept. In either case, you can think of the neurotransmitter as "carrying the message." However, this messenger

Continued

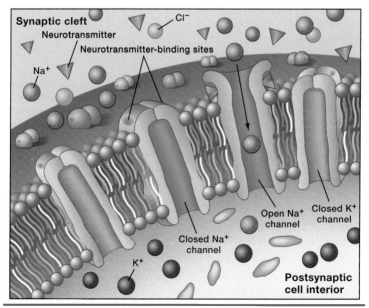

Figure 3-6 Direct stimulation of postsynaptic receptor. Some neurotransmitters, such as acetylcholine, initiate nerve signals by binding directly to one or both neurotransmitter-binding sites on the stimulus-gated ion channel. Such binding causes the channel to change its shape to an open position. When the neurotransmitter is removed, the channel again closes.

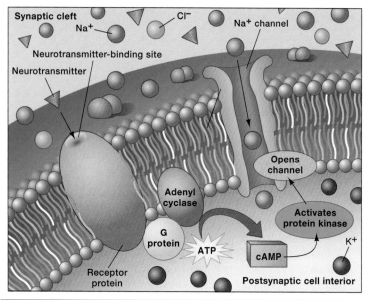

Figure 3-7 Second-messenger stimulation of postsynaptic receptor.
Norepinephrine (NE) and many other neurotransmitters initiate nerve signals indirectly by binding to a receptor linked to a G protein that changes shape to activate the enzyme adenylate cyclase, which in turn catalyzes the conversion of adenosine triphosphate (ATP) to cyclic adenosine monophosphate (cAMP). cAMP is a second messenger that induces a change in the shape of a stimulus-gated channel. (Compare with Figure 3-6.)

Field Notes—cont'd

can get it inside the cell—it's blocked from directly entering the cell. Therefore it has to send the signal inside the cell—which is the process of signal transduction. It is sort of like when a person delivers a message to someone in a building, but can't actually get into the building—they have to get the message inside some other way.

The direct approach to signal transduction (see Figure 3-6) is like when a person is delivering a message such as, "Open the sodium door, please." However, it can't get inside to the sodium door operator, so the messenger presses the intercom button on the outside of the sodium door and says to the operator inside, "Open the sodium door, please." That's pretty direct—it uses a mechanism that's pretty much built into the doorway itself. Of course, the message could have been, "Close the sodium door, please," or "Open the potassium door, please." It depends on the specific neurotransmitter and the specific receptor/transduction mechanism.

Continued on page 182

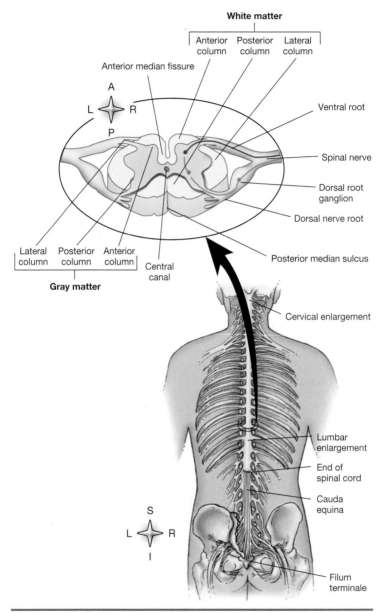

Figure 3-8 Spinal cord. The inset illustrates a transverse section of the spinal cord shown in the broader view.

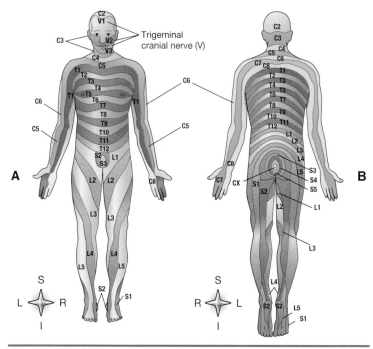

Figure 3-9 Dermatome distribution of spinal nerves. A, The front of the body's surface. **B,** The back of the body's surface. Cervical segments and spinal nerves *(C)*; thoracic segments and spinal nerves *(T)*; lumbar segments and spinal nerves *(L)*; sacral segments and spinal nerves *(S)*.

Field Notes—cont'd

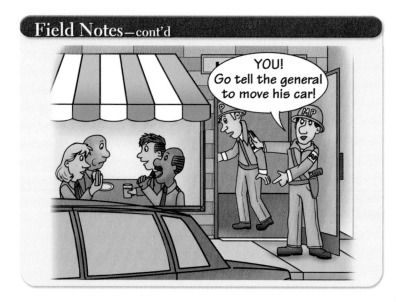

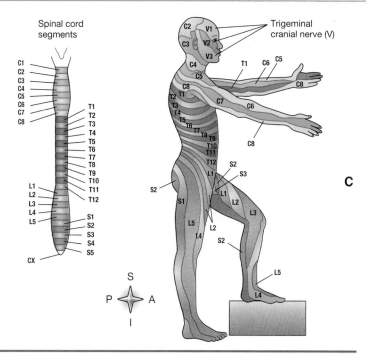

Figure 3-9—cont'd Dermatome distribution of spinal nerves. C, The side of the body's surface. The inset shows the segments of the spinal cord associated with each of the spinal nerves associated with the sensory dermatomes shown.

Field Notes—cont'd

The second-messenger approach (see Figure 3-7) is only one of several such systems—but one that serves as a good example. Here, it's like a messenger who gets to the building to deliver the message, "Open the sodium door, please" and can't get in. Therefore the messenger hands off the message to someone inside the building (maybe through a mail slot). Then the message is handed off to a second messenger on the inside who sees that the message is passed along into a system that will eventually get the message to the sodium door operator.

The second-messenger approach seems unnecessarily complex. Such complexity is valuable, however, because its gives more opportunities to the cell (or outside agents) to modify (adjust) the message before it gets to its final destination. In other words, it allows the operation of "dimmer switches" that allow us to increase or decrease certain events triggered in the cell.

Table 3-3	Examples of Neurotransmitters

NEURO-TRANSMITTER	LOCATION*	FUNCTION*
Small-Molecule Transmitters		
Acetylcholine	Junctions with motor effectors (muscles, glands); many parts of brain	Excitatory or inhibitory; involved in memory
Amines MONOAMINES		
Serotonin	Several regions of the central nervous system (CNS)	Mostly inhibitory; involved in moods and emotions, sleep
Histamine	Brain	Mostly excitatory; involved in emotions and regulation of body temperature and water balance
CATECHOLAMINES		
Dopamine	Brain, autonomic system	Mostly inhibitory; involved in emotions and moods and in regulating motor control
Epinephrine	Several areas of the CNS and in the sympathetic division of the autonomic nervous system (ANS)	Excitatory or inhibitory; acts as a hormone when secreted by sympathetic neuro-secretory cells of the adrenal gland
Norepinephrine (NE)	Several areas of the CNS and in the sympathetic division of the ANS	Excitatory or inhibitory; regulates sympathetic effectors; in brain, involved in emotional responses
Amino Acids		
Glutamate (glutamic acid)	CNS	Excitatory; most common excitatory neurotransmitter in CNS

Table 3-3	Examples of Neurotransmitters—cont'd	
NEURO-TRANSMITTER	**LOCATION***	**FUNCTION***
Gamma-aminobutyric acid (GABA)	Brain	Inhibitory; most common inhibitory neurotransmitter
Glycine	Spinal cord	Inhibitory; most common inhibitory neurotransmitter in brain
Large-Molecule Transmitters		
Neuropeptides		
Vasoactive intestinal peptide (VIP)	Brain; some ANS and sensory fibers; retina; gastro-intestinal (GI) tract	Function in nervous system uncertain
Cholecystokinin (CCK)	Brain, retina	Function in nervous system uncertain
Substance P	Brain, spinal cord, sensory pain pathways; GI tract	Mostly excitatory; transmits pain information
Enkephalins	Several regions of CNS; retina; intestinal tract	Mostly inhibitory; act like opiates to block pain
Endorphins	Several regions of CNS; retina; intestinal tract	Mostly inhibitory; act like opiates to block pain
Other Small Molecules		
Nitric oxide (NO)	Uncertain	May be a signal from postsynaptic to presynaptic neuron

*These are examples only; most of these neurotransmitters are also found in other locations and many have additional functions.

Table 3-4 — Major Ascending Tracts of Spinal Cord

NAME	FUNCTION
Lateral spinothalamic	Pain, temperature, and crude touch opposite side
Anterior spinothalamic	Crude touch and pressure
Fasciculi gracilis and cuneatus	Discriminating touch and pressure sensations, including vibration, stereognosis, and two-point discrimination; also conscious kinesthesia
Anterior and posterior spinocerebellar	Unconscious kinesthesia
Spinotectal	Touch related to visual reflexes

*Location of cell bodies of neurons from which axons of tract arise.
†Structure in which axons of tract terminate.

Table 3-5 — Major Descending Tracts of Spinal Cord

NAME	FUNCTION
Lateral corticospinal (or crossed pyramidal)	Voluntary movement, contraction of individual or small groups of muscles, particularly those moving hands, fingers, feet, and toes of opposite side
Anterior corticospinal (direct pyramidal)	Same as lateral corticospinal except mainly muscles of same side
Reticulospinal	Maintain posture during movement
Rubrospinal	Coordination of body movement and posture
Tectospinal	Head and neck movement during visual reflexes
Vestibulospinal	Coordination of posture and balance

*Location of cell bodies of neurons from which axons of tract arise.
†Structure in which axons of tract terminate.

LOCATION	ORIGIN*	TERMINATION†
Lateral white columns	Posterior gray column opposite side	Thalamus
Anterior white columns	Posterior gray column opposite side	Thalamus
Posterior white columns	Spinal ganglia same side	Medulla
Lateral white columns	Anterior or posterior gray column	Cerebellum
Lateral white columns	Posterior gray columns	Superior colliculus (midbrain)

LOCATION	ORIGIN*	TERMINATION†
Lateral white columns	Motor areas or cerebral cortex opposite side from tract location in cord	Lateral or anterior gray columns
Anterior white columns	Motor cortex but on same side as location in cord	Lateral or anterior gray column
Anterior white columns	Reticular formation (midbrain, pons, and medulla)	Anterior gray columns
Lateral white columns	Red nucleus (of midbrain)	Anterior gray columns
Anterior white columns	Superior colliculus (midbrain)	Medulla and anterior gray columns
Anterior white columns	Vestibular nucleus (pons, medulla)	Anterior gray columns

Table 3-6	Spinal Nerves and Peripheral Branches		
SPINAL NERVES	**PLEXUSES FORMED FROM ANTERIOR RAMI**	**SPINAL NERVE BRANCHES FROM PLEXUSES**	**PARTS SUPPLIED**
Cervical 1 2 3 4	Cervical plexus	Lesser occipital Greater auricular Cutaneous nerve of neck Supraclavicular nerves Branches to muscles	Sensory to back of head, front of neck, and upper part of shoulder; motor to numerous neck muscles
Cervical 5 6 7 8	Brachial plexus	Phrenic nerve Suprascapular and dorsoscapular Thoracic nerves, medial and lateral branches Long thoracic nerve	Diaphragm Superficial muscles* of scapula Pectoralis major and minor Serratus anterior
Thoracic (dorsal) 1 2 3 4 5 6 7 8 9 10 11 12	No plexus formed; branches run directly to intercostal muscles and skin of thorax	Thoracodorsal Subscapular Axillary (circumflex) Musculocutaneous Ulnar	Latissimus dorsi Subscapular and teres major muscles Deltoid and teres minor muscles and skin over deltoid Muscles of front of arm (biceps brachii, coracobrachialis, and brachialis) and skin on outer side of forearm Flexor carpi ulnaris and part of flexor digitorum profundus; some of muscles of hand; sensory to medial side of hand, little finger, and medial half of fourth finger

*Although nerves to muscles are considered motor, they do contain some sensory fibers that transmit proprioceptive impulses.

Table 3-6		Spinal Nerves and Peripheral Branches—cont'd	
SPINAL NERVES	**PLEXUSES FORMED FROM ANTERIOR RAMI**	**SPINAL NERVE BRANCHES FROM PLEXUSES**	**PARTS SUPPLIED**
		Median	Rest of muscles of front of forearm and hand; sensory to skin of palmar surface of thumb, index, and middle fingers
		Radial	Triceps muscle and muscles of back of forearm; sensory to skin of back of forearm and hand
		Medial cutaneous	Sensory to inner surface of arm and forearm
Lumbar 1 2 3 4 5	Lumbosacral plexus	Iliohypogastric Ilioinguinal (sometimes fused with iliohypogastric)	Sensory to anterior abdominal wall Sensory to anterior abdominal wall and external genitalia; motor to muscles of abdominal wall
Sacral 1 2 3 4 5		Genitofemoral	Sensory to skin of external genitalia and inguinal region
		Lateral femoral cutaneous	Sensory to outer side of thigh
		Femoral	Motor to quadriceps, sartorius, and iliacus muscles; sensory to front of thigh and medial side of lower leg (saphenous nerve)

†Sensory fibers from the tibial and peroneal nerves unite to form the medial cutaneous (or sural) nerve that supplies the calf of the leg and the lateral surface of the foot. In the thigh the tibial and common peroneal nerves are usually enclosed in a single sheath to form the sciatic nerve, the largest nerve in the body with a width of approximately 3/4 inch (2 cm). About two thirds of the way down the posterior part of the thigh, it divides into its component parts. Branches of the sciatic nerve extend into the hamstring muscles.

Continued

Table 3-6		Spinal Nerves and Peripheral Branches—cont'd	
SPINAL NERVES	**PLEXUSES FORMED FROM ANTERIOR RAMI**	**SPINAL NERVE BRANCHES FROM PLEXUSES**	**PARTS SUPPLIED**
		Obturator	Motor to adductor muscles of thigh
		Tibial† (medial popliteal)	Motor to muscles of calf of leg; sensory to skin of calf of leg and sole of foot
Coccygeal 1	Coccygeal plexus	Common peroneal (lateral popliteal)	Motor to evertors and dorsiflexors of foot; sensory to lateral surface of leg and dorsal surface of foot
		Nerves to hamstring muscles	Motor to muscles of back of thigh
		Gluteal nerves	Motor to buttock muscles and tensor fasciae latae
		Posterior femoral cutaneous	Sensory to skin of buttocks, posterior surface of thigh, and leg
		Pudendal nerve	Motor to perineal muscles; sensory to skin of perineum

Table 3-7	Major Regions of the Brain
REGION	**GENERAL FUNCTIONS**
Brain Stem	
Medulla oblongata	Two-way conduction pathway between the spinal cord and higher brain centers; integration/regulation in cardiac, respiratory, and vasomotor control centers
Pons	Two-way conduction pathway; influences regulation of breathing
Midbrain	Two-way conduction pathway; regulation of auditory and visual reflexes

Table 3-7	Major Regions of the Brain—cont'd

REGION	GENERAL FUNCTIONS
Diencephalon	
Hypothalamus	Regulation of body temperature, water balance, sleep-cycle control, appetite, sexual arousal, pituitary, and endocrine function
Thalamus	Sensory relay station from body areas to the cerebral cortex; some motor relaying out of cortex; emotions and alerting/arousal mechanism
Pineal gland	Monitor external light conditions and signals the body with the timekeeping hormone melatonin
Cerebellum	Coordination of skilled muscle activity; posture and equilibrium; monitors body position and other sensory information; generally assists cerebral functions
Cerebrum	Conscious perception and thinking, willed movements, memory, problem-solving, processing sensory and motor data, language, other higher-order functions

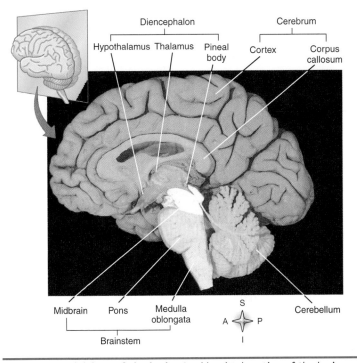

Figure 3-10 Divisions of the brain. A midsagittal section of the brain reveals features of its major divisions.

Table 3-8   Structure and Function of the Cranial Nerves

| Nerve* | SENSORY FIBERS | | |
	Receptors	Cell Bodies	Termination
I **Olfactory**	Nasal mucosa	Nasal mucosa	Olfactory bulbs (new relay of neurons to olfactory cortex)
II **Optic**	Retina (proprioceptive) Skin and mucosa of head, teeth	Retina	Nucleus in thalamus (lateral geniculate) some fibers terminate in superior colliculus of midbrain
III **Oculomotor**	External eye muscles except superior oblique and lateral rectus	Trigeminal ganglion	Midbrain (oculo-motor nucleus)
IV **Trochlear**	Superior oblique (proprioceptive)	Trigeminal ganglion	Midbrain
V **Trigeminal**	Skin and mucosa of head, teeth	Trigeminal ganglion	Pons (sensory nucleus)
VI **Abducens**	Lateral rectus (proprioceptive)	Trigeminal ganglion	Pons
VII **Facial**	Taste buds of anterior two thirds of tongue	Geniculate ganglion	Medulla (nucleus solitarius)
VIII Vestibulocochlear			
Vestibular branch	Semicircular canals and vestibule (utricle and saccule)	Vestibular ganglion	Pons and medulla (vestibular nuclei)
Cochlear or auditory branch	Organ of Corti in cochlear duct	Spiral ganglion	Pons and medulla (cochlear nuclei)

	sensory (afferent); motor (efferent)	
MOTOR FIBERS		
Cell Bodies	**Termination**	**Functions**
		Sense of smell
		Vision
Midbrain (oculomotor nucleus)	External eye muscles except superior oblique and lateral rectus; autonomic fibers terminate in ciliary ganglion and then to ciliary and iris muscles	Eye movements, regulation of size of pupil, accommodation (for near vision), **proprioception (muscle sense)**
Midbrain	Superior oblique muscle of eye	Eye movements, **proprioception**
Pons (motor nucleus)	Muscles of mastication	**Sensations of head and face,** chewing movements, **proprioception**
Pons	Lateral rectus muscle of eye	Abduction of eye, **proprioception**
Pons	Superficial muscles of face and scalp; autonomic fibers to salivary and lacrimal glands	Facial expressions, secretion of saliva and tears, **taste**
		Balance or equilibrium sense
		Hearing

Continued

Table 3-8   Structure and Function of the Cranial Nerves—cont'd

| Nerve* | SENSORY FIBERS | | |
	Receptors	Cell Bodies	Termination
IX **Glossopharyngeal**	Pharynx; taste receptors of buds and other posterior one third of tongue	Jugular and petrous ganglia	Medulla (nucleus solitarius)
	Carotid sinus and carotid body	Jugular and petrous ganglia	Medulla (respiratory and vasomotor centers)
X **Vagus**	Pharynx, larynx, carotid body, and thoracic and abdominal viscera	Jugular and nodose ganglia	Medulla (nucleus solitarius), pons (nucleus of fifth cranial nerve)
XI **Accessory**	Trapezius and sternocleidomastoid (proprioceptive)	Upper, cervical ganglia	Spinal cord
XII **Hypoglossal**	Tongue muscles (proprioceptive)	Trigeminal ganglion	Medulla (hypoglossal nucleus)

*The first letter of the words in the following sentence are the first letters of the name of the cranial nerves, in the correct order. Many anatomy students find that using this sentence, or one like it, helps in memorizing the names and numbers of the cranial nerves. It is "**O**n **O**ld **O**lympus' **T**iny **T**ops, **A** **F**riendly **V**iking **G**rew **V**ines **A**nd **H**ops."

| □ sensory (afferent); □ motor (efferent) |

MOTOR FIBERS

Cell Bodies	Termination	Functions
Medulla (nucleus ambiguus)	Muscles of pharynx	Sensations of tongue, swallowing movements, secretion of saliva, aid in reflex control of blood pressure and respiration
Medulla at junction of pons (nucleus salivatorius)	Otic ganglion and then to parotid salivary gland	
Medulla (dorsal motor nucleus)	Ganglia of vagal plexus and then to muscles of pharynx, larynx, and autonomic fibers to thoracic and abdominal viscera	Sensations and movements of organs supplied (e.g., slows heart, increases peristalsis, and contracts muscles for voice production)
Medulla (dorsal motor nucleus of vagus and nucleus ambiguus) Anterior gray column of first five or six cervical segments of spinal cord	Muscles of thoracic and abdominal viscera (autonomic) and pharynx and larynx Trapezius and sternocleidomastoid muscle	Shoulder movements, turning movements of head, movements of viscera, voice production, proprioception
Medulla (hypoglossal nucleus)	Muscles of tongue and throat	

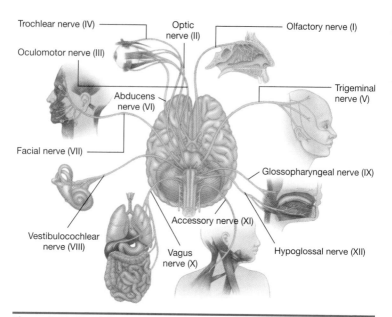

Figure 3-11 Cranial nerves. Ventral surface of the brain showing attachment of the cranial nerves.

Table 3-9	Comparison of Somatic Motor and Autonomic Pathways	
FEATURE	**SOMATIC MOTOR PATHWAYS**	**AUTONOMIC EFFERENT PATHWAYS**
Direction of information flow	Efferent	Efferent
Number of neurons between central nervous system (CNS) and effector	One (somatic motor neuron)	Two (preganglionic and postganglionic)
Myelin sheath present	Yes	Preganglionic: yes Postganglionic: no
Location of peripheral fibers	Most cranial nerves and all spinal nerves	Most cranial nerves and all spinal nerves
Effector innervated	Skeletal muscle (voluntary)	Smooth and cardiac muscle, glands (involuntary)
Neurotransmitter	Acetylcholine	Acetylcholine or norepinephrine (NE)

Table 3-10 Comparison of Structural Features of the Sympathetic and Parasympathetic Pathways

NEURONS	SYMPATHETIC	PARASYMPATHETIC
Preganglionic Neurons		
Dendrites and cell bodies	In lateral gray columns of thoracic and first four lumbar segments of spinal cord	In nuclei of brainstem and in lateral gray columns of sacral segments of cord
Axons	In anterior roots of spinal nerves to spinal nerves (thoracic and first four lumbar), to and through white rami to terminate in sympathetic ganglia at various levels or to extend through sympathetic ganglia, to and through splanchnic nerves to terminate in collateral ganglia	From brainstem nuclei through cranial nerve III to ciliary ganglion From nuclei in pons through cranial nerve VII to sphenopalatine or submaxillary ganglion From nuclei in medulla through cranial nerve IX to otic ganglion or through cranial nerves X and XI to cardiac and celiac ganglia, respectively
Distribution	Short fibers from central nervous system (CNS) to ganglion	Long fibers from CNS to ganglion
Neurotransmitter	Acetylcholine	Acetylcholine
Ganglia	Sympathetic chain ganglia (22 pairs); collateral ganglia (celiac, superior, and inferior mesenteric)	Terminal ganglia (in or near effector)
Postganglionic Neurons		
Dendrites and cell bodies	In sympathetic and collateral ganglia	In parasympathetic ganglia (e.g., ciliary, sphenopalatine, submaxillary, otic, cardiac, celiac) located in or near visceral effector organs
Receptors	Cholinergic (nicotinic)	Cholinergic (nicotinic)
Axons	In autonomic nerves and plexuses that innervate thoracic and abdominal viscera and blood vessels in these cavities In gray rami to spinal nerves, to smooth muscle of skin blood vessels and hair follicles, and to sweat glands	In short nerves to various visceral effector organs
Distribution	Long fibers from ganglion to widespread effectors	Short fibers from ganglion to single effector
Neurotransmitter	Norepinephrine (NE) (many); acetylcholine (few)	Acetylcholine

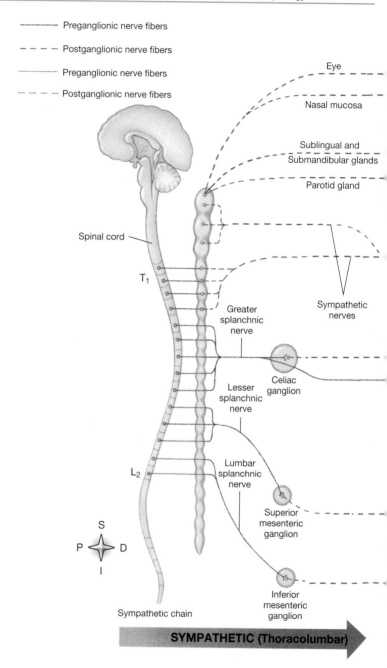

Preganglionic nerve fibers
Postganglionic nerve fibers
Preganglionic nerve fibers
Postganglionic nerve fibers

Eye

Nasal mucosa

Sublingual and
Submandibular glands

Parotid gland

Spinal cord

T_1

Greater
splanchnic
nerve

Sympathetic
nerves

Celiac
ganglion

Lesser
splanchnic
nerve

Lumbar
splanchnic
nerve

L_2

Superior
mesenteric
ganglion

S

P   D

I

Inferior
mesenteric
ganglion

Sympathetic chain

SYMPATHETIC (Thoracolumbar)

Figure 3-12 Major autonomic motor conduction paths. The left side of
the diagram *(orange)* shows the outline of the sympathetic motor pathways.
The right side of the diagram *(green)* shows the major parasympathetic
motor pathways. Notice that conduction from the spinal cord to any visceral

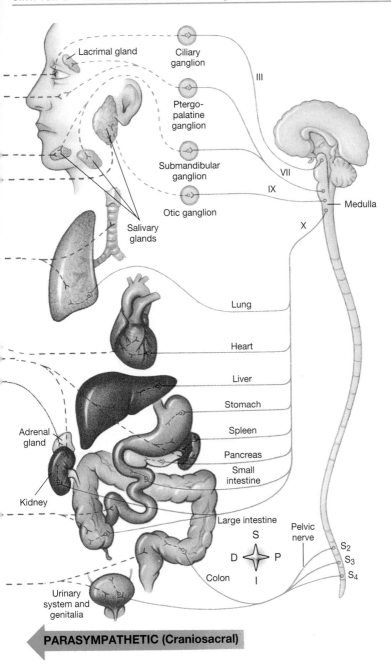

Lacrimal gland

Ciliary ganglion

III

Ptergo-palatine ganglion

Submandibular ganglion

VII

IX

Otic ganglion

Medulla

Salivary glands

X

Lung

Heart

Liver

Stomach

Spleen

Pancreas

Small intestine

Adrenal gland

Kidney

Large intestine

Pelvic nerve

S

D   ✦   P

I

Colon

S_2

S_3

S_4

Urinary system and genitalia

PARASYMPATHETIC (Craniosacral)

effector requires a relay of at least two autonomic motor neurons—a pre-ganglionic *(solid line)* and a postganglionic neuron *(broken line)*. Notice also that many of the representative autonomic effectors *(center of diagram)* are dually innervated *(by both autonomic motor divisions)*.

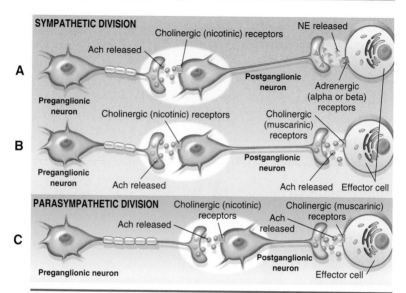

Figure 3-13 **Locations of neurotransmitters and receptors of the autonomic nervous system.** In all pathways, preganglionic fibers are cholinergic, secreting acetylcholine *(Ach)*, which stimulates nicotinic receptors in the postganglionic neuron. **A,** Most sympathetic postganglionic fibers are adrenergic, secreting norepinephrine *(NE)*, thus stimulating alpha- or beta-adrenergic receptors. **B,** A few sympathetic postganglionic fibers are cholinergic, stimulating muscarinic receptors in effector cells. **C,** All parasympathetic postganglionic fibers are cholinergic, stimulating muscarinic receptors in effector cells.

Table 3-11	Autonomic Functions	
AUTONOMIC EFFECTOR	**EFFECT OF SYMPATHETIC STIMULATION (NEURO-TRANSMITTER: NOREPI-NEPHRINE [NE] UNLESS OTHERWISE STATED)**	**EFFECT OF PARASYMPA-THETIC STIMULATION (NEUROTRANSMITTER: ACETYLCHOLINE)**
Cardiac Muscle	Increased rate and strength of contraction (beta receptors)	Decreased rate and strength of contraction
Smooth Muscle of Blood Vessels		
Skin blood vessels	Constriction (alpha receptors)	No effect
Skeletal muscle blood vessels	Dilation (beta receptors)	No effect

Table 3-11 Autonomic Functions—cont'd

AUTONOMIC EFFECTOR	EFFECT OF SYMPATHETIC STIMULATION (NEUROTRANSMITTER: NOREPINEPHRINE [NE] UNLESS OTHERWISE STATED)	EFFECT OF PARASYMPATHETIC STIMULATION (NEUROTRANSMITTER: ACETYLCHOLINE)
Coronary blood vessels	Constriction (alpha receptors) Dilation (beta receptors)	Dilation
Abdominal blood vessels	Constriction (alpha receptors)	No effect
Blood vessels of external genitals	Constriction (alpha receptors)	Dilation of blood vessels causing erection
Smooth Muscle of Hollow Organs and Sphincters		
Bronchioles	Increased peristalsis	Constriction
Digestive tract, except sphincters	Relaxation	Increased peristalsis
Sphincters of digestive tract	Contraction	Relaxation
Urinary bladder	Relaxation	Contraction
Urinary sphincters	Relaxation	Relaxation
Reproductive ducts	Constriction	Relaxation
Eye		
Iris	Contraction of radial muscle; dilated pupil Relaxation; accommodates for far vision	Contraction of circular muscle; constricted pupil Contraction; accommodates for near vision
Ciliary (pilomotor muscles)	Contraction produces goose pimples, or piloerection (alpha receptors)	No effect
Glands		
Sweat	Increased sweat (neurotransmitter, acetylcholine)	No effect
Lacrimal	No effect	Increased secretion of tears

Continued

Table 3-11   Autonomic Functions—cont'd

AUTONOMIC EFFECTOR	EFFECT OF SYMPATHETIC STIMULATION (NEURO-TRANSMITTER: NOR-EPINEPHRINE [NE] UNLESS OTHERWISE STATED)	EFFECT OF PARASYMPA-THETIC STIMULATION (NEUROTRANSMITTER: ACETYLCHOLINE)
Digestive (salivary, gastric)glands	Decreased secretion of saliva; not known for others	Increased secretion of saliva
Pancreas, including islets	Decreased secretion	Increased secretion of pancreatic juice and insulin
Liver	Increased glycogenolysis (beta receptors); increased blood sugar level	No effect
Adrenal medulla*	Increased epinephrine secretion	No effect

*Sympathetic preganglionic axons terminate in contact with secreting cells of the adrenal medulla. Thus the adrenal medulla functions, to quote someone's descriptive phrase, as a "giant sympathetic postganglionic neuron."

Table 3-12   Summary of the Sympathetic "Fight-or-Flight" Reaction

RESPONSE	ROLE IN PROMOTING ENERGY USED BY SKELETAL MUSCLES
Increased heart rate	Increased rate of blood flow, thus increased delivery of oxygen (O_2) and glucose to skeletal muscles
Increased strength of cardiac muscle contraction	Increased rate of blood flow, thus increased delivery of O_2 and glucose to skeletal muscles
Dilation of coronary vessels of the heart	Increased delivery of O_2 and nutrients to cardiac muscle to sustain increased rate and strength of heart contractions
Dilation of blood vessels in skeletal muscles	Increased delivery of O_2 and nutrients to skeletal muscles
Constriction of blood vessels in digestive and other organs	Shunting of blood to skeletal muscles to increase O_2 and glucose delivery

Table 3-12	Summary of the Sympathetic "Fight-or-Flight" Reaction—cont'd	

RESPONSE	ROLE IN PROMOTING ENERGY USED BY SKELETAL MUSCLES
Contraction of spleen and other blood reservoirs	More blood discharged into general circulation, causing increased delivery of O_2 and glucose to skeletal muscles
Dilation of respiratory airways	Increased loading of O_2 into blood
Increased rate and depth of breathing	Increased loading of O_2 into blood
Increased sweating	Increased dissipation of heat generated by skeletal muscle activity
Increased conversion of glycogen into glucose	Increased amount of glucose available to skeletal muscles

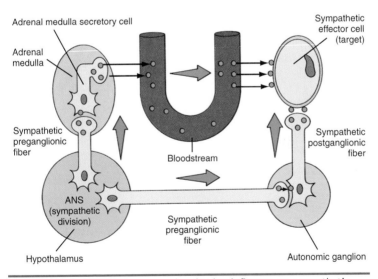

Figure 3-14 Combined nervous and endocrine influence on sympathetic effectors during the "fight-or-flight" response. A sympathetic center in the hypothalamus sends efferent impulses through preganglionic fibers. Some preganglionic fibers synapse with postganglionic fibers that deliver norepinephrine (NE) across a synapse with the effector cell. Other preganglionic fibers synapse with postganglionic neurosecretory cells in the adrenal medulla. These neurosecretory cells secrete epinephrine and NE into the bloodstream, where they travel to the target cells (sympathetic effectors) to produce the stress response. Epinephrine in the bloodstream prolongs and enhances the more immediate but short-lived effects of NE released at the effector.

Table 3-13 Classification of Somatic Sensory Receptors

BY STRUCTURE	BY LOCATION AND TYPE	BY ACTIVATION STIMULUS	BY SENSATION OR FUNCTION
Free Nerve Endings			
Nociceptors	Both extero-ceptors and viscerocep-tors—most body tissues	Almost any noxious stimulus; temperature change; mechanical	Pain, tempera-ture, itch, tickle
Merkel discs	Exteroceptors	Light pressure, mechanical	Discriminative touch
Root hair plexuses	Exteroceptors	Hair move-ment, mechanical	Sense of "deflection" type move-ment of hair
Encapsulated Nerve Endings			
Touch and Pressure Receptors			
Meissner's corpuscle	Exteroceptors; epidermis, hairless skin	Light pressure, mechanical	Touch; low-frequency vibration

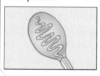

Table 3-13   Classification of Somatic Sensory Receptors—cont'd

BY STRUCTURE	BY LOCATION AND TYPE	BY ACTIVATION STIMULUS	BY SENSATION OR FUNCTION
Krause's corpuscle	Mucous membranes	Mechanical	Touch; low-frequency vibration
Ruffini's corpuscle	Dermis of skin, exteroceptors	Mechanical	Crude and persistent touch
Pacinian corpuscle	Dermis of skin, joint capsules	Deep pressure, mechanical	Deep pressure; high-frequency vibration; stretch
Stretch Receptors			
Muscle spindles	Skeletal muscle	Stretch, mechanical	Sense of muscle length
Golgi tendon receptors	Musculo-tendinous junction	Force of contraction and tendon stretch, mechanical	Sense of muscle tension

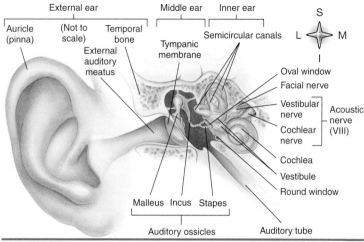

Figure 3-15 The ear. External, middle, and inner ear. (Anatomic structures are not drawn to scale.) The bony labyrinth is the hard outer wall of the entire inner ear and includes semicircular canals, vestibule, and cochlea. Within the bony labyrinth is the membranous labyrinth (not visible), which is surrounded by perilymph and filled with endolymph. Structures in the vestibule have receptors that detect changes in head position and send sensory impulses through the vestibular nerve to the brain. Receptors in the cochlea detect sound vibrations in the inner ear fluids. The vestibular and cochlear nerves join to form the eighth cranial nerve.

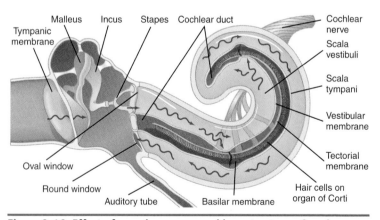

Figure 3-16 Effect of sound waves on cochlear structures. Sound waves strike the tympanic membrane and cause it to vibrate. This causes the membrane of the oval window to vibrate, which causes the perilymph in the bony labyrinth of the cochlea and the endolymph in the membranous labyrinth of the cochlea, or cochlear duct, to move. This movement of endolymph causes the basilar membrane to vibrate, which in turn stimulates hair cells on the organ of Corti to transmit nerve impulses along the cranial nerve. Eventually, nerve impulses reach the auditory cortex and are interpreted as sound.

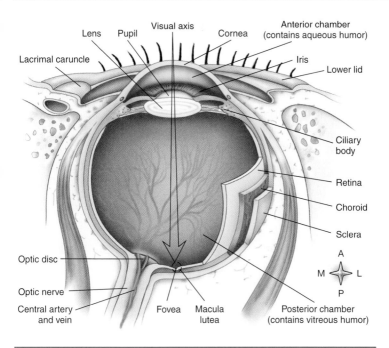

Figure 3-17 Horizontal section through the right eyeball. The eye is viewed from above.

Table 3-14	Coats of the Eyeball		
POSTERIOR LOCATION	**PORTION**	**ANTERIOR PORTION**	**CHARACTERISTICS**
Outer coat (sclera)	Sclera proper	Cornea	Protective fibrous coat, cornea transparent, rest of coat white and opaque
Middle coat (choroid)	Choroid proper	Ciliary body, suspensory ligament, iris (pupil is hole in iris); lens suspended in suspensory ligament	Vascular, pigmented coat
Inner coat (retina)	Retina	No anterior portion	Nervous tissue; rods and cones (receptors for second cranial nerve) located in retina

Table 3-15   Cavities of the Eye

CAVITY	DIVISIONS	LOCATION	CONTENTS
Anterior	Anterior chamber	Anterior to iris and posterior to cornea	Aqueous humor
	Posterior chamber	Posterior to iris and anterior to lens	Aqueous humor
Posterior	None	Posterior to lens	Vitreous humor

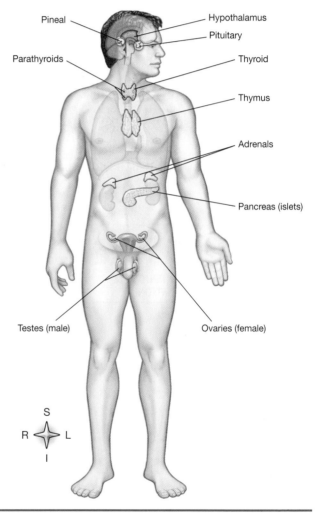

Figure 3-18 Locations of some major endocrine glands.

Table 3-16	Names and Locations of Some Major Endocrine Glands

NAME	LOCATION
Hypothalamus	Cranial cavity (brain)
Pituitary gland	Cranial cavity
Pineal gland	Cranial cavity (brain)
Thyroid gland	Neck
Parathyroid glands	Neck
Thymus	Mediastinum
Adrenal glands	Abdominal cavity (retroperitoneal)
Pancreatic islets	Abdominal cavity (pancreas)
Ovaries	Pelvic cavity
Testes	Scrotum
Placenta	Pregnant uterus

Table 3-17	Comparison of Features of the Endocrine System and Nervous System

FEATURE	ENDOCRINE SYSTEM	NERVOUS SYSTEM
Overall function	Regulation of effectors to maintain homeostasis	Regulation of effectors to maintain homeostasis
Control by regulatory feedback loops	Yes (endocrine reflexes)	Yes (nervous reflexes)
Effector tissues	Endocrine effectors: virtually all tissues	Nervous effectors: muscle and glandular tissue only
Effector cells	Target cells (throughout the body)	Postsynaptic cells (in muscle and glandular tissue only)
Chemical messenger	Hormone	Neurotransmitter
Cells that secrete the chemical messenger	Glandular epithelial cells or neurosecretory cells (modified neurons)	Neurons

Continued

Table 3-17	Comparison of Features of the Endocrine System and Nervous System—cont'd	
FEATURE	**ENDOCRINE SYSTEM**	**NERVOUS SYSTEM**
Distance traveled (and method of travel) by chemical messenger	Long (by way of circulating blood)	Short (across a microscopic synapse)
Location of receptor in effector cell	On the plasma membrane or within the cell	On the plasma membrane
Characteristics of regulatory effects	Slow to appear, long-lasting	Appear rapidly, short lived

Field Notes

Cable or Satellite?

Comparing nervous regulation and endocrine regulation as in Table 3-17 is important for understanding the overall regulatory scheme of the body. Often, they are considered together as a single *neuroendocrine* system.

An analogy that can be useful in understanding the difference between these two styles of regulation in the body is based on television signals. As with TV signals, both endocrine and nervous signals are generated in a central location (or several central locations) and then sent out to individuals (individual effector cells in this case).

How a person gets a TV signal can vary: cable, local broadcast, satellite. Nervous regulation is more like cable TV because each effector cell has to be individually "hooked up"—that is, connected to an efferent nerve pathway. Of course, you need a cable decoder box too. In a nervous effector cell (postsynaptic cell), that takes the form of specific receptors and associated signal transduction mechanisms.

Endocrine regulation is similar to satellite TV—you don't have to have a direct line. Hormones are like satellites because they are simply sent out everywhere. If you have the right equipment such as a satellite dish and decoder, then you can receive the signals. If you

Field Notes—cont'd

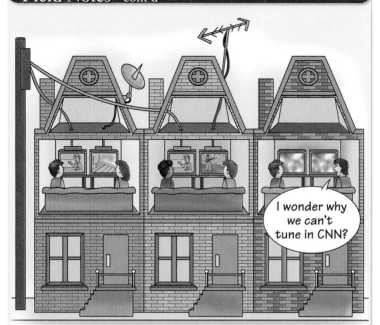

don't have the equipment, then you're still being bombarded with signals—you just can't receive or interpret them. Similarly, all cells have contact with hormones—they move through the entire bloodstream. However, only target cells—that is, those cells with the correct receptors for the specific hormone—actually hear the message and respond to it.

We can also consider local regulation here (paracrine regulation). Local regulation is more like local broadcast TV, rather than cable or satellite. That's because the signals are sent by radio waves to a local community and can travel only a relatively short distance. In other words, you can only receive the signal locally. The TV waves, like local regulatory molecules, can only spread out over the local area. If you have the right equipment, however, such as an antenna and tuner, then you can receive these signals. As with satellite signals, if you don't have the equipment, the signals are still bombarding you— you just can't receive or interpret them. Only those cells with the correct receptors (or some way to respond) for a specific local regulator are affected by the local signal.

Table 3-18   Chemical Classification of Selected Hormones[*]

CATEGORY	SUBCATEGORY	HORMONE
Steroid		Cortisol
		Aldosterone
		Estrogen
		Progesterone
		Testosterone
Nonsteroid	Protein	Growth hormone (GH)
		Prolactin (PRL)
		Parathyroid hormone (PTH)
		Calcitonin (CT)
		Adrenocorticotropic hormone (ACTH)
		Insulin
		Glucagon
	Glycoprotein	Follicle-stimulating hormone (FSH)
		Luteinizing hormone (LH)
		Thyroid-stimulating hormone (TSH)
		Human chorionic gonadotropin (hCG)
	Peptide	Antidiuretic hormone (ADH) Arginine vasopressin (AVP)
		Oxytocin (OT)
		Somatostatin (SS)
		Thyrotropin-releasing hormone (TRH)
		Gonadotropin-releasing hormone (GnRH)
		Atrial natriuretic hormone (ANH) Atrial natriuretic peptide (ANP)
	Amino acid derivative	Norepinephrine (NE)
	Amine	Noradrenaline (NA)
		Epinephrine Adrenaline
		Melatonin
	Iodinated amino	Tetraiodothyronine (T_4) Thyroxine
		Triiodothyronine (T_3)

*Does not include prostaglandins and related compounds.

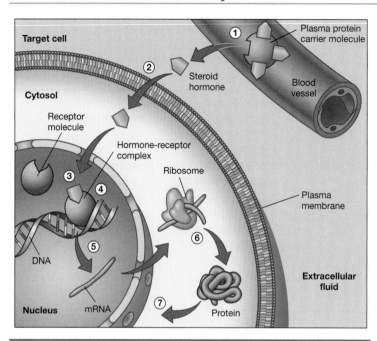

Figure 3-19 Steroid hormone mechanism. According to the mobile-receptor model, lipid-soluble steroid hormone molecules detach from a carrier protein *(1)* and pass through the plasma membrane *(2)*. The hormone molecules then pass into the nucleus where they bind with a mobile receptor to form a hormone-receptor complex *(3)*. This complex then binds to a specific site on a DNA molecule *(4)*, triggering transcription of the genetic information encoded there *(5)*. The resulting mRNA molecule moves to the cytosol, where it associates with a ribosome, initiating synthesis of a new protein *(6)*. This new protein—usually an enzyme or channel protein—produces specific effects in the target cell *(7)*. Some steroid hormones also have additional secondary effects such as influencing signal transduction pathways at the plasma membrane. (Steroid hormones may have additional effects similar to those shown in Figure 3-20.)

Table 3-19	Comparison of Steroid and Nonsteroid Hormones	
CHARACTERISTIC	**STEROID HORMONES**	**NONSTEROID HORMONES***
Chemical structure	Lipid	One or more amino acids, sometimes with added sugar groups
Stored in secretory cell	No	Yes; stored in secretory vesicles before release

Continued

Table 3-19	Comparison of Steroid and Nonsteroid Hormones—cont'd	
CHARACTERISTIC	**STEROID HORMONES**	**NONSTEROID HORMONES***
Interaction with plasma membrane	No; simple diffusion through plasma membrane and into target	Yes; binds to specific plasma membrane receptor cell
Receptor	Mobile receptor in cytoplasm or nucleus	Embedded in plasma membrane
Action	Regulates gene activity (transcription of new proteins that eventually produce effects in the cell)	Triggers signal transduction cascade, producing internal second messengers that trigger rapid effects in the target cell
Response time	One hour to several days	Several seconds to a few minutes

*Some nonsteroidal hormones derived from amino acids (such as thyroid hormones T3 and T4) have gene-activating actions similar to steroid hormones.

Table 3-20	Prostaglandins and Related Hormones		
HORMONE	**SOURCE**	**TARGET**	**PRINCIPAL ACTION**
Prostaglandins (PGs)	Many diverse tissues of the body	Local cells within the source tissue	Diverse local (paracrine and autocrine) effects such as regulation of inflammation and muscle contraction in blood vessels
Thromboxanes (TXs)	Platelets	Other platelets; muscles in blood vessel walls	Increases stickiness of platelets; promotes blood clotting; causes constriction of blood vessels
Leukotrienes	Several types of white blood cell (WBC; leukocyte)	Local cells of various types	Produce local inflammation triggered by allergens, including constriction of airways (as in asthma) and other inflammatory responses

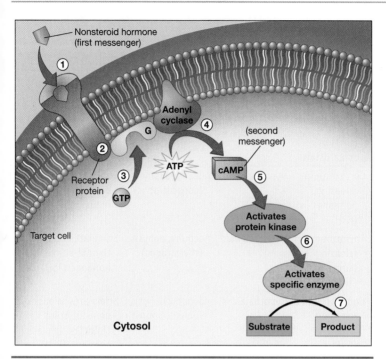

Figure 3-20 Example of a second-messenger mechanism. A nonsteroidal hormone (first messenger) binds to a fixed receptor in the plasma membrane of the target cell *(1)*. The hormone-receptor complex activates the G protein *(2)*. The activated G protein reacts with glomerulotubular protein (GTP), which in turn activates the membrane-bound enzyme adenyl cyclase *(3)*. Adenyl cyclase removes phosphates from adenosine triphosphate (ATP,) converting it to cyclic adenosine monophosphate (cAMP) (second messenger) *(4)*. cAMP activates or inactivates protein kinases *(5)*. Protein kinases activate specific intracellular enzymes *(6)*. These activated enzymes then influence specific cellular reactions, thus producing the target cell's response to the hormone *(7)*. (Some nonsteroidal hormones, such as thyroid hormones T3 and T4, have effects similar to those seen in Figure 3-19.)

Table 3-21 Hormones of the Hypothalamus

HORMONE	SOURCE	TARGET	PRINCIPAL ACTION
Growth hormone–releasing hormone (GRH)	Hypothalamus	Adenohypophysis (somatotrophs)	Stimulates secretion (release) of growth hormone

Continued

Table 3-21	Hormones of the Hypothalamus—cont'd		
HORMONE	**SOURCE**	**TARGET**	**PRINCIPAL ACTION**
Growth hormone–inhibiting hormone (GIH) or somatostatin	Hypothalamus	Adenohypophysis (somatotrophs)	Inhibits secretion of growth hormone
Corticotropin-releasing hormone (CRH)	Hypothalamus	Adenohypophysis (corticotrophs)	Stimulates release of adrenocorticotropic hormone (ACTH)
Thyrotropin-releasing hormone (TRH)	Hypothalamus	Adenohypophysis (thyrotrophs)	Stimulates release of thyroid-stimulating hormone (TSH)
Gonadotropin-releasing hormone (GnRH)	Hypothalamus	Adenohypophysis (gonadotrophs)	Stimulates release of gonadotropins (follicle-stimulating hormone [FSH] and luteinizing hormone [LH])
Prolactin-releasing hormone (PRH)	Hypothalamus	Adenohypophysis (corticotrophs)	Stimulates secretion of prolactin
Prolactin-inhibiting hormones (PIH)	Hypothalamus	Adenohypophysis (corticotrophs)	Inhibits secretion of prolactin

Table 3-22	Hormones of the Pituitary Gland		
HORMONE	**SOURCE**	**TARGET**	**PRINCIPAL ACTION**
Growth hormone (GH) (somatotropin [STH])	Adenohypophysis (somatotrophs)	General	Promotes growth by stimulating protein anabolism and fat mobilization
Prolactin (PRL) (lactogenic hormone)	Adenohypophysis (lactotrophs)	Mammary glands (alveolar secretory cells)	Promotes milk secretion

Table 3-22 — Hormones of the Pituitary Gland—cont'd

HORMONE	SOURCE	TARGET	PRINCIPAL ACTION
Thyroid-stimulating hormone (TSH)*	Adenohypophysis (thyrotrophs)	Thyroid gland	Stimulates development and secretion in the thyroid gland
Adrenocortico-tropic hormone (ACTH)*	Adenohypophysis (corticotrophs)	Adrenal cortex	Promotes development and secretion in the adrenal cortex
Follicle-stimulating hormone (FSH)*	Adenohypophysis (gonadotrophs)	Gonads (primary sex organs)	*Female:* Promotes development of ovarian follicle; simulates estrogen secretion *Male:* Promotes development of testis; stimulates sperm production
Luteinizing hormone (LH)*	Adenohypophysis (gonadotrophs)	Gonads	*Female:* Triggers ovulation; promotes development of corpus luteum *Male:* Stimulates production of testosterone
Antidiuretic hormone (ADH) or arginine vasopressin (AVP)	Neurohypophysis	Kidney	Promotes water retention by kidney tubules; raises blood pressure by stimulating muscles in walls of small arteries
Oxytocin (OT)	Neurohypophysis	Uterus and mammary glands	Stimulates uterine contractions; stimulates ejection of milk into ducts of mammary glands

*Tropic hormones.

Table 3-23   Hormones of the Thyroid and Parathyroid Glands

HORMONE	SOURCE	TARGET	PRINCIPAL ACTION
Triiodothyronine (T_3)	Thyroid gland (follicular cells)	General	Increases rate of metabolism
Tetraiodo-thyronine (T_4) or thyroxine	Thyroid gland (follicular cells)	General	Increases rate of metabolism (usually converted to T_3 first)
Calcitonin (CT)	Thyroid gland (parafollicular cells)	Bone tissue	Increases calcium (Ca^{++}) storage in bone, lowering blood Ca^{++} levels
Parathyroid hormone (PTH) or para-thormone	Parathyroid glands	Bone tissue and kidney	Increases Ca^{++} removal from storage in bone and produces the active form of vitamin D in the kidneys, increasing absorption of Ca^{++} by intestines and increasing blood Ca^{++} levels

Table 3-24   Hormones of the Adrenal Glands

HORMONE	SOURCE	TARGET	PRINCIPAL ACTION
Aldosterone	Adrenal cortex (zona glomerulosa)	Kidney	Stimulates kidney tubules to conserve sodium, which in turn triggers the release of antidiuretic hormone (ADH) and the resulting conservation of water by the kidney
Cortisol (hydro-cortisone)	Adrenal cortex (zona fasciculata)	General	Influences metabolism of food molecules; in large amounts, it has an antiinflammatory effect
Adrenal androgens	Adrenal cortex (zona reticularis)	Sex organs, other effectors	Exact role uncertain, but may support sexual function

Table 3-24   Hormones of the Adrenal Glands—cont'd

HORMONE	SOURCE	TARGET	PRINCIPAL ACTION
Adrenal estrogens	Adrenal cortex (zona reticularis)	Sex organs	Thought to be physiologically insignificant
Epinephrine (adrenaline)	Adrenal medulla	Sympathetic effectors	Enhances and prolongs the effects of the sympathetic division of the autonomic nervous system (ANS)
Norepinephrine (NE)	Adrenal medulla	Sympathetic effectors	Enhances and prolongs the effects of the sympathetic division of the ANS

Table 3-25   Hormones of the Pancreatic Islets

HORMONE	SOURCE	TARGET	PRINCIPAL ACTION
Glucagon	Pancreatic islets (alpha [a] cells or A cells)	General	Promotes movement of glucose from storage and into the blood
Insulin	Pancreatic islets (beta [b] cells or B cells)	General	Promotes movement of glucose out of the blood and into cells
Somatostatin	Pancreatic islets (delta [D] cells or D cells)	Pancreatic cells and other effectors	Can have general effects in the body but primary role seems to be regulation of secretion of other pancreatic hormones
Pancreatic polypeptide	Pancreatic islets (pancreatic polypeptide [PP] or F cells)	Intestinal cells and other effectors	Exact function uncertain but seems to influence absorption in the digestive tract

Table 3-26	Examples of Additional Hormones of the Body		
HORMONE	**SOURCE**	**TARGET**	**PRINCIPAL ACTION**
Cholecalciferol (vitamin D_3)	Skin, liver, and kidney (in progressive steps)	Intestines, bones, most other tissues	Promotes calcium (Ca^{++}) absorption from food, regulates mineral balance in bones, regulates growth and differentiation of many cell types
Dehydroepian-drosterone (DHEA)	Adrenal gland, testis, ovary, other tissues	Converted to other hormones	Eventually converted to estrogens and/or testosterone (see Figure 6-5)
Melatonin	Pineal gland	Timekeeping tissues of the nervous system	Helps "set" the biologic clock mechanisms of the body by signaling light changes during the day, month, and seasons; may help induce sleep
Testosterone	Testis (small amounts in adrenal and ovary)	Sperm-producing tissues of testis, muscles, other tissues	Stimulates sperm production, stimulates growth and maintenance of male sexual characteristics, promotes muscle growth
Estrogen, including estradiol (E_2) and estrone	Ovary and placenta (small amounts in adrenal and testis)	Uterus, breasts, other tissues	
Progesterone	Ovary and placenta	Uterus, mammary glands, other tissues	Helps maintain proper conditions for pregnancy
Human chorionic gonadotropin (hCG)	Placenta	Ovary	Stimulates secretion of estrogen and progesterone during pregnancy

Table 3-26 Examples of Additional Hormones of the Body—cont'd

HORMONE	SOURCE	TARGET	PRINCIPAL ACTION
Human placental lactogens (HPLs)	Placenta	Mammary glands, pancreas, and other tissues	Promote development of mammary glands during pregnancy; help regulate energy balance in fetus
Relaxin	Placenta	Uterus, joints	Inhibits uterine contractions during pregnancy and softens pelvic joints to facilitate childbirth
Thymosins and thymopoietins	Thymus gland	Certain lymphocytes (type of white blood cell [WBC])	Stimulate development of T lymphocytes, which are involved in immunity
Gastrin	Stomach mucosa	Exocrine glands of stomach	Triggers increased gastric juice secretion
Secretin	Intestinal mucosa	Stomach and pancreas	Increases alkaline secretions of the pancreas and slows emptying of stomach
Cholecystokinin (CCK)	Intestinal mucosa	Gallbladder and pancreas	Triggers the release of bile from gallbladder and enzymes from the pancreas
Ghrelin	Stomach mucosa	Hypothalamus; other diverse tissues	Stimulates hypothalamus to boost appetite; affects energy balance in various tissues
Atrial natriuretic hormone (ANH) and other atrial natriuretic peptides (ANPs)	Heart muscle	Kidney	Promotes loss of sodium from body into urine, thus promoting water loss from the body and a resulting decrease in blood volume and pressure

Continued

Table 3-26 Examples of Additional Hormones of the Body—cont'd

HORMONE	SOURCE	TARGET	PRINCIPAL ACTION
Inhibins	Ovary	Adenohypophysis (anterior pituitary)	Inhibit secretion of FSH by the anterior pituitary, thus helping to regulate the female reproductive cycle
Leptin	Adipose tissue	Hypothalamus; other diverse tissues	Affects energy balance, perhaps as a signal of how much fat is stored; affects various immune, neuroendocrine, and developmental functions throughout body
Resistin	Adipose tissue and macrophages	Liver and other tissues	Reduces sensitivity to insulin (a pancreatic islet hormone); thus increases blood glucose levels

CHAPTER FOUR

Transportation and Defense

TOPICS

Cardiovascular system, lymphatic system, immunity

Table 4-1	Classes of Blood Cells		
CELL TYPE	**DESCRIPTION**	**FUNCTION**	**LIFE SPAN**
Erythrocyte	7 μm in diameter; concave disk shape; entire cell stains pale pink; no nucleus	Transportation of respiratory gases (oxygen [O_2] and carbon dioxide [CO_2])	105 to 120 days
Neutrophil	12-15 μm in diameter; spheric shape; multilobed nucleus; small, pink-purple–staining cytoplasmic granules	Cellular defense—Phagocytosis of small pathogenic microorganisms	Hours to 3 days
Basophil	11-14 μm in diameter; spheric shape; generally two-lobed nucleus; large purple-staining cytoplasmic granules	Secretes heparin (anticoagulant) and histamine (important in inflammatory response)	Hours to 3 days

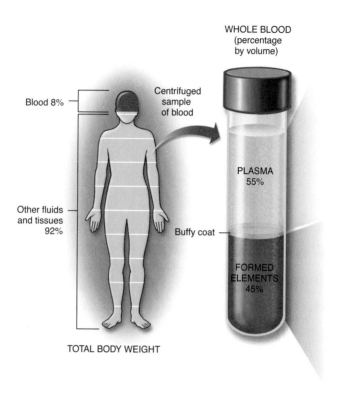

Figure 4-1 **Composition of whole blood.** Approximate values for the components of blood in a normal adult.

Table 4-1	Classes of Blood Cells—cont'd		
CELL TYPE	**DESCRIPTION**	**FUNCTION**	**LIFE SPAN**
Eosinophil	10-12 μm in diameter; spheric shape; generally two-lobed nucleus; large orange-red–staining cytoplasmic granules	Cellular defense—Phagocytosis of large pathogenic microorganisms such as protozoa and parasitic worms; releases antiinflammatory substances in allergic reactions	10 to 12 days

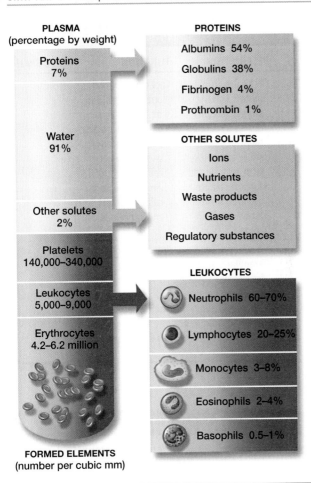

PLASMA
(percentage by weight)

Proteins 7%

Water 91%

Other solutes 2%

Platelets 140,000–340,000

Leukocytes 5,000–9,000

Erythrocytes 4.2–6.2 million

FORMED ELEMENTS
(number per cubic mm)

PROTEINS

Albumins 54%

Globulins 38%

Fibrinogen 4%

Prothrombin 1%

OTHER SOLUTES

Ions

Nutrients

Waste products

Gases

Regulatory substances

LEUKOCYTES

Neutrophils 60–70%

Lymphocytes 20–25%

Monocytes 3–8%

Eosinophils 2–4%

Basophils 0.5–1%

Table 4-1	Classes of Blood Cells—cont'd		
CELL TYPE	**DESCRIPTION**	**FUNCTION**	**LIFE SPAN**
Lymphocyte	6-9 μm in diameter; spheric shape; round (single lobe) nucleus; small lymphocytes have scant cytoplasm	Humoral defense— Secretes antibodies; involved in immune system response and regulation	Days to years

Continued

Table 4-1	Classes of Blood Cells—cont'd		
CELL TYPE	**DESCRIPTION**	**FUNCTION**	**LIFE SPAN**
Monocyte	12-17 μm in diameter; spheric shape; nucleus generally kidney bean or "horseshoe" shaped with convoluted surface; ample cytoplasm often "steel blue" in color	Capable of migrating out of the blood to enter tissue spaces as a macrophage (an aggressive phagocytic cell capable of ingesting bacteria, cellular debris, and cancerous cells)	Months
Platelet	2-5 μm in diameter; irregularly shaped fragments; cytoplasm contains very small pink-staining granules	Releases clot-activating substances and helps in formation of actual blood clot by forming platelet "plugs"	7 to 10 days

Table 4-2	Differential Count of White Blood Cells	
	DIFFERENTIAL COUNT*	
CLASS	**NORMAL RANGE (%)**	**TYPICAL VALUE (%)**
Neutrophils	65 to 75	65
Eosinophils	2 to 5	3
Basophils	$1/2$ to 1	1
Lymphocytes (large and small)	20 to 25	25
Monocytes	3 to 8	6
Total	100	100

*In any differential count, the sum of the percentages of the different kinds of white blood cells (WBCs) must, of course, total 100%.

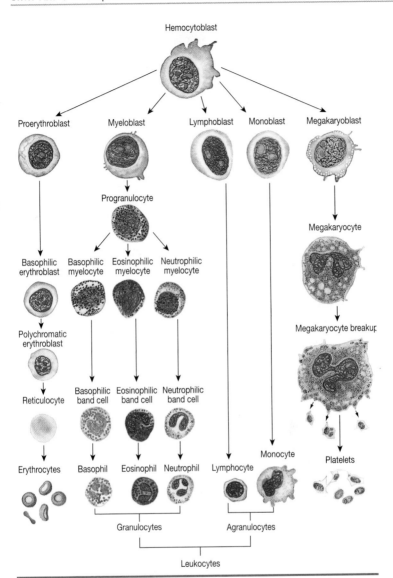

Figure 4-2 Formation of blood cells. The hematopoietic stem cell serves as the original stem cell from which all formed elements of the blood are derived. Note that all five precursor cells, which ultimately produce the different components of the formed elements, are derived from the hematopoietic stem cell called a hemocytoblast.

Field Notes

Field Marks

Recall from the special section on the anatomy and physiology (A&P) laboratory course (see page 42) that field marks are used by naturalists to quickly distinguish between two similar species of plant or animal (or whatever) while out on a field trip. Field guides often highlight these distinguishing characteristics with arrows or some other way to tell you what to look for. For many animals, such as birds, you may only have a moment to look at them. If all you remember is that *it was big and yellow,* then you probably won't be able to accurately identify it. However, if your field guide shows that the several kinds of big yellow birds can be distinguished by the color of their beaks—you can figure that out quickly and accurately.

This method works wonderfully for many structures of the body, too, as we have seen. Tissues, bones and bone features, muscles, and

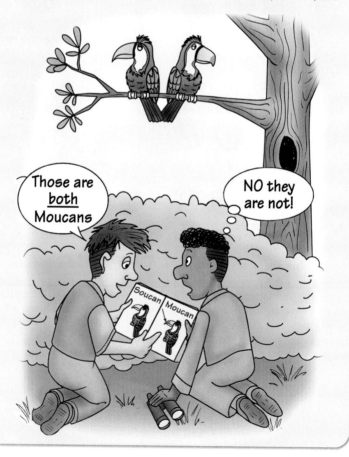

Field Notes—cont'd

so on, can all be easily distinguished once you've discovered their one or two unique characteristics—their field marks.

This *field mark method* is especially helpful when trying to distinguish between different types of white blood cells (WBCs, leukocytes) when doing a differential WBC count—that is, a count of how many of each type of WBC you have in your sample (see Table 4-2).

Using Table 4-1, make your own *field guide to the WBCs.* Enlarge the table on a color photocopier and cut out the blood cell images— or, even better, draw your own color sketches of them. Then put arrows on the figures where each cell type differs from other similar cell types. Then write a brief notation, such as "two-lobed nucleus" to tell what the field mark arrow points to or how to distinguish it.

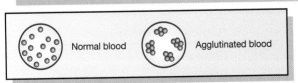

Recipient's blood		Reactions with donor's blood			
RBC antigens	Plasma antibodies	Donor type O	Donor type A	Donor type B	Donor type AB
None (Type O)	Anti-A Anti-B				
A (Type A)	Anti-B				
B (Type B)	Anti-A				
AB (Type AB)	(None)				

Normal blood   Agglutinated blood

Figure 4-3 ABO blood types. Results of different combinations of donor and recipient blood. The left columns show the recipient's blood characteristics, and the top row shows the donor's blood type.

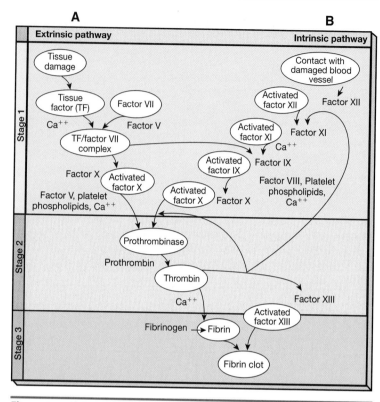

Figure 4-4 Clot formation. A, Extrinsic clotting pathway. *Stage 1:* Damaged tissue releases tissue factor, which with factor VII and calcium ions activates factor X. Activated factor X, factor V, phospholipids, and calcium ions form prothrombinase. *Stage 2:* Prothrombin is converted to thrombin by prothrombinase. *Stage 3:* Fibrinogen is converted to fibrin by thrombin. Fibrin forms a clot. **B,** Intrinsic clotting pathway. *Stage 1:* Damaged vessels cause activation of factor XII. Activated factor XII activates factor XI, which activates factor IX. Factor IX, along with factor VIII and platelet phospholipids, activates factor X. Activated factor X, factor V, phospholipids, and calcium ions form prothrombinase. *Stages 2* and *3* take the same course as the extrinsic clotting pathway.

Table 4-3	Coagulation Factors—Standard Nomenclature and Synonyms
FACTOR	**COMMON SYNONYM(S)**
Factor I	Fibrinogen
Factor II	Prothrombin
Factor III	Thromboplastin
	Thrombokinase

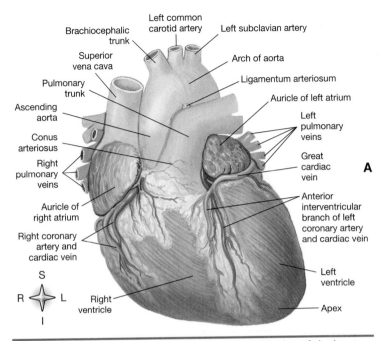

Figure 4-5 The heart and central vessels. A, Anterior view of the heart and great vessels. *Continued*

Table 4-3	Coagulation Factors—Standard Nomenclature and Synonyms—cont'd
FACTOR	**COMMON SYNONYM(S)**
Factor IV	Calcium
Factor V	Proaccelerin Labile factor
Factor VI (now obsolete)	None in use
Factor VII	Serum prothrombin conversion accelerator (SPCA)
Factor VIII	Antihemophilic globulin (AHG) Antihemophilic factor (AHF)
Factor IX	Plasma thromboplastin component (PTC), Christmas factor
Factor X	Stuart factor
Factor XI	Plasma thromboplastin antecedent (PTA)
Factor XII	Hageman factor
Factor XIII	Fibrin-stabilizing factor

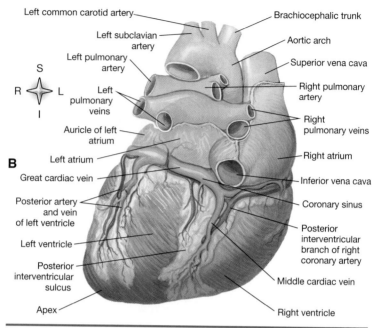

Figure 4-5—cont'd **The heart and central vessels. B,** Posterior view of the heart and great vessels.

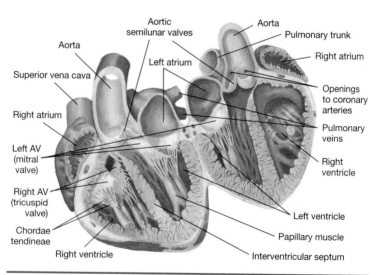

Figure 4-6 **Interior of the heart.** This illustration shows the heart as it would appear if it were cut along a frontal plane and opened like a book. The front portion of the heart lies to the reader's right; the back portion of the heart lies to the reader's left. The four chambers of the heart—two atria and two ventricles—are easily seen.

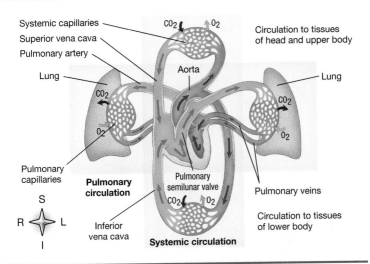

Figure 4-7 Blood flow through the circulatory system. In the pulmonary circulatory route, blood is pumped from the right side of the heart to the gas-exchange tissues of the lungs. In the systemic circulation, blood is pumped from the left side of the heart to all other tissues of the body.

Table 4-4	Structure of Blood Vessels		
TYPE OF VESSEL	**TUNICA INTIMA (ENDOTHELIUM)**	**TUNICA MEDIA (SMOOTH MUSCLE; ELASTIC CONNECTIVE TISSUE)**	**TUNICA EXTERNA (FIBROUS TYPE OF VESSEL CONNECTIVE TISSUE)**
Arteries	Smooth lining	Allows constriction and dilation of vessels; thicker than in veins; muscle innervated by autonomic fibers	Provides flexible support that resists collapse or injury; thicker than in veins; thinner than tunica media
Veins	Smooth lining with semilunar valves to ensure one-way flow	Allows constriction and dilation of vessels; thinner than in arteries; muscle innervated by autonomic fibers	Provides flexible support that resists collapse or injury; thinner than in arteries; thicker than tunica media
Capillaries	Makes up entire wall of capillary; thinness permits ease of transport across vessel wall	Absent	Absent

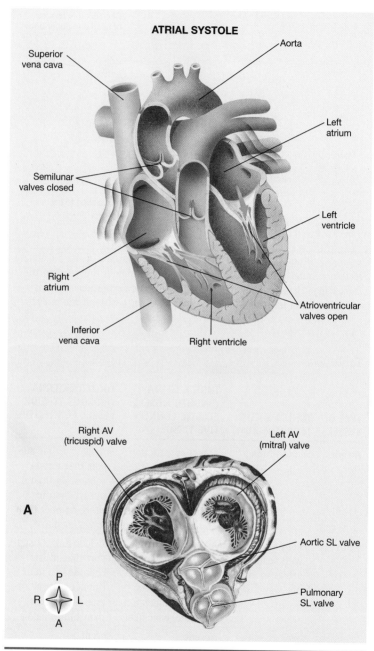

Figure 4-8 Heart action. A, During atrial systole (contraction), cardiac muscle in the atrial wall contracts, forcing blood through the atrioventricular *(AV)* valves and into the ventricles. Bottom illustration shows superior view of all four valves (atria removed), with semilunar *(SL)* valves closed and AV valves open.

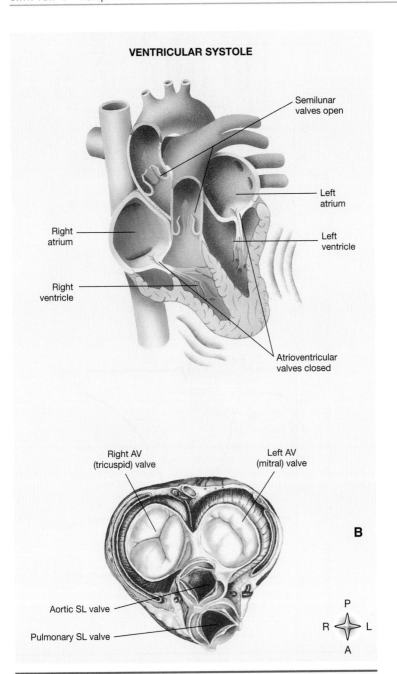

VENTRICULAR SYSTOLE

Semilunar valves open

Left atrium

Right atrium

Left ventricle

Right ventricle

Atrioventricular valves closed

Right AV (tricuspid) valve

Left AV (mitral) valve

B

Aortic SL valve

Pulmonary SL valve

P

R — L

A

Figure 4-8—cont'd Heart action. B, During ventricular systole that follows, the AV valves close, and blood is forced out of the ventricles through the semilunar valves and into the arteries. Bottom illustration shows superior view of SL valves open and AV valves closed.

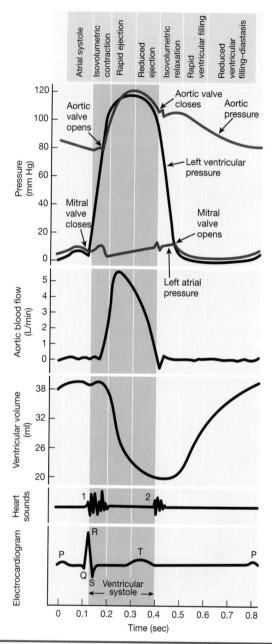

Figure 4-9 Composite chart of heart function. This chart is a composite of several diagrams of heart function (cardiac pumping cycle, blood pressure, blood flow, volume, heart sounds, and electrocardiogram [ECG]), all adjusted to the same time scale.

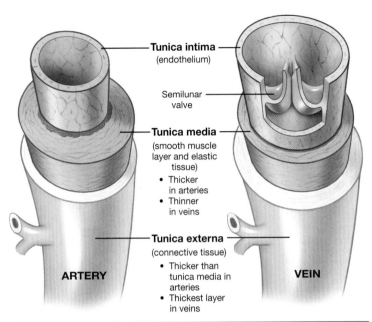

Figure 4-10 Artery and vein. Schematic drawings of an artery and a vein show comparative thicknesses of the three layers: the outer layer (or tunica externa), the muscle layer (or tunica media), and the tunica intima made of endothelium. Note that the muscle and outer layer are much thinner in veins than in arteries and that veins have valves.

Table 4-5	Major Systemic Arteries	
ARTERY*	**REGION SUPPLIED**	
Ascending Aorta		
Coronary arteries	Myocardium	
Arch of Aorta		
Brachiocephalic (innominate)	Head and upper extremity	
Right subclavian	Head, upper extremity	
Right vertebral†	Spinal cord, brain	
Right axillary (continuation of subclavian)	Shoulder, chest, axillary region	
Right brachial (continuation of axillary)	Arm and hand	

*Branches of each artery are indented below its name.
†See figures for branches of the artery.

Continued on page 240

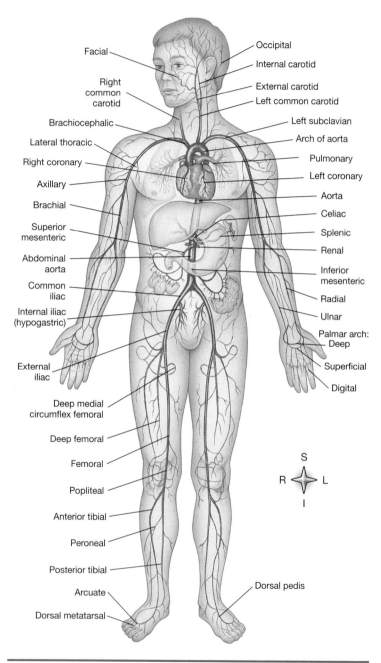

Figure 4-11 Principal arteries of the body.

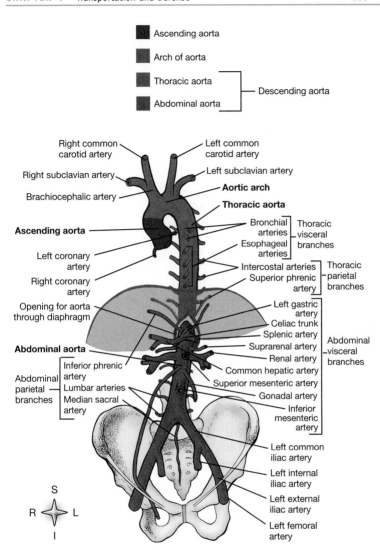

Figure 4-12 Divisions and primary branches of the aorta. *Anterior view:* The aorta is the main systemic artery, serving as a trunk from which other arteries branch. Blood is conducted from the heart first through the ascending aorta; then the arch of the aorta; then through the thoracic and abdominal segments of the descending aorta. Note the designation of visceral and parietal branches in the thoracic and abdominal aortic divisions. Table 4-5 and the schematics showing branches of the aortic divisions are intended to assist you in interpreting chapter illustrations of arterial vessels.

Table 4-5 Major Systemic Arteries—cont'd

ARTERY*	REGION SUPPLIED
Right radial	Lower arm and hand (lateral)
Right ulnar	Lower arm and hand (medial)
Superficial and deep palmar arches (formed by anastomosis of branches of radial and ulnar)	Hand and fingers
Digital	Fingers
Right common carotid	Head and neck
Right internal carotid[†]	Brain, eye, forehead, nose
Right external carotid[†]	Thyroid, tongue, tonsils, ear
Left subclavian	Head and upper extremity
Left vertebral[†]	Spinal cord, brain
Left axillary (continuation of subclavian)	Shoulder, chest, axillary region
Left brachial (continuation of axillary)	Arm and hand
Left radial	Lower arm and hand (lateral)
Left ulnar	Lower arm and hand (medial)
Superficial and deep palmar arches (formed by anastomosis of branches of radial and ulnar)	Hand and fingers
Digital	Fingers
Left common carotid	Head and neck
Left internal carotid[†]	Brain, eye, forehead, nose
Left external carotid[†]	Thyroid, tongue, tonsils, ear
Descending Thoracic Aorta	
Visceral branches	Thoracic viscera
Bronchial	Lungs, bronchi
Esophageal	Esophagus
Parietal branches	Thoracic walls
Intercostal	Lateral thoracic walls (rib cage)
Superior phrenic	Superior surface of diaphragm

*Branches of each artery are indented below its name.
[†]See figures for branches of the artery.

Table 4-5	Major Systemic Arteries—cont'd

ARTERY*	REGION SUPPLIED
Descending Abdominal Aorta	
Visceral branches	Abdominal viscera
Celiac artery (trunk)	Abdominal viscera
Left gastric	Stomach, esophagus
Common hepatic	Liver
Splenic	Spleen, pancreas, stomach
Superior mesenteric	Pancreas, small intestine, colon
Inferior mesenteric	Descending colon, rectum
Suprarenal	Adrenal (suprarenal) gland
Renal	Kidney
Ovarian	Ovary, uterine tube, ureter
Testicular	Testis, ureter
Parietal branches	Walls of abdomen
Inferior phrenic	Inferior surface of diaphragm, adrenal gland
Lumbar	Lumbar vertebrae and muscles of back
Median sacral	Lower vertebrae
Common iliac (formed by terminal branches of aorta)	Pelvis, lower extremity
External iliac	Thigh, leg, foot
Femoral (continuation of external iliac)	Thigh, leg, foot
Popliteal (continuation of femoral)	Leg, foot
Anterior tibial	Leg, foot
Posterior tibial	Leg, foot
Plantar arch (formed by anastomosis of branches of anterior and posterior tibial arteries)	Foot, toes
Digital	Toes
Internal iliac	Pelvis
Visceral branches	Pelvic viscera
Middle rectal	Rectum
Vaginal	Vagina, uterus
Uterine	Uterus, vagina, uterine tube, ovary

Continued

Table 4-5	Major Systemic Arteries—cont'd

ARTERY*	REGION SUPPLIED
Parietal branches	Pelvic wall and external regions
Lateral sacral	Sacrum
Superior gluteal	Gluteal muscles
Obturator	Pubic region, hip joint, groin
Internal pudendal	Rectum, external genitals, floor of pelvis
Inferior gluteal	Lower gluteal region, coccyx, upper thigh

*Branches of each artery are indented below its name.
†See text and figures for branches of the artery.

Table 4-6	Major Systemic Veins

VEIN*	REGION DRAINED
Superior Vena Cava	Head, neck, thorax, upper extremity
BRACHIOCEPHALIC (innominate)	Head, neck, upper extremity
Internal jugular (continuation of sigmoid sinus)	Brain
Lingual	Tongue, mouth
Superior thyroid	Thyroid, deep face
Facial	Superficial face
Sigmoid sinus (continuation of transverse sinus/direct tributary of internal jugular)	Brain, meninges, skull
Superior and inferior petrosal sinuses	Anterior brain, skull
Cavernous sinus	Anterior brain, skull
Ophthalmic veins	Eye, orbit
Transverse sinus (direct tributary of sigmoid sinus)	Brain, meninges, skull
Occipital sinus	Inferior, central region of cranial cavity
Straight sinus	Central region of brain, meninges
Inferior sagittal sinus	Central region of brain, meninges
Superior sagittal (longitudinal) **sinus**	Superior region of cranial cavity
External jugular	Superficial, posterior head, neck
Subclavian (continuation of axillary or direct tributary of brachiocephalic)	Axilla, lower extremity
Axillary (continuation of basilic or direct tributary of subclavian)	Axilla, lower extremity

*Tributaries of each vein are indented below its name; deep veins are printed in dark blue, and superficial veins are printed in light blue.

Table 4-6 Major Systemic Veins—cont'd

VEIN*	REGION DRAINED
Cephalic	Lateral and lower arm, hand
Brachial	Deep arm
Radial	Deep lateral forearm
Ulnar	Deep medial forearm
Basilic (direct tributary of axillary)	Medial and lower arm, hand
Median cubital (basilic) (formed by anastomosis of cephalic and basilic)	Arm, hand
Deep and superficial **palmar venous arches** (formed by anastomosis of cephalic and basilic)	Hand
Digital	Fingers
AZYGOS (anastomoses with right ascending lumbar)	Right posterior wall of thorax and abdomen, esophagus, bronchi, pericardium, mediastinum
Hemiazygos (anastomoses with left renal)	Left inferior posterior wall of thorax and abdomen, esophagus, mediastinum
Accessory hemiazygos	Left superior posterior wall of thorax
Inferior Vena Cava	Lower trunk and extremity
PHRENIC	Diaphragm
Hepatic portal system	Upper abdominal viscera
Hepatic veins (continuations of liver venules and sinusoids and, ultimately, the hepatic portal vein)	Liver
Hepatic portal vein	Gastrointestinal (GI) organs, pancreas, spleen, gallbladder
Cystic	Gallbladder
Gastric	Stomach
Splenic	Spleen
Inferior mesenteric	Descending colon, rectum
Pancreatic	Pancreas
Superior mesenteric	Small intestine, most of colon
Gastroepiploic	Stomach
RENAL	Kidneys
Suprarenal	Adrenal (suprarenal) gland
Left ovarian	Left ovary
Left testicular	Left testis
Left ascending lumbar (anastomoses with hemiazygos)	Left lumbar region

Continued

Table 4-6   Major Systemic Veins—cont'd

VEIN*	REGION DRAINED
Right ovarian	Right ovary
Right testicular	Right testis
Right ascending lumbar (anastomoses with azygos)	Right lumbar region
Common iliac (continuation of external iliac; common iliacs unite to form inferior vena cava)	Lower extremity
External iliac (continuation of femoral or direct tributary of common iliac)	Thigh, leg, foot
Femoral (continuation of popliteal or direct tributary of external iliac)	Thigh, leg, foot
Popliteal	Leg, foot
Posterior tibial	Deep posterior leg
Medial and lateral plantar	Sole of foot
Fibular (peroneal) (continuation of anterior tibial)	Lateral and anterior leg, foot
Anterior tibial	Anterior leg, foot
Dorsal veins of foot	Anterior (dorsal) foot, toes
Small (external, short) saphenous	Superficial posterior leg, lateral foot
Great (internal, long) saphenous	Superficial medial and anterior thigh, leg, foot
Dorsal veins of foot	Anterior (dorsal) foot, toes
Dorsal venous arch	Anterior (dorsal) foot, toes
Digital	Toes
INTERNAL ILIAC	Pelvic region

*Tributaries of each vein are indented below its name; deep veins are printed in dark blue, and superficial veins are printed in light blue.

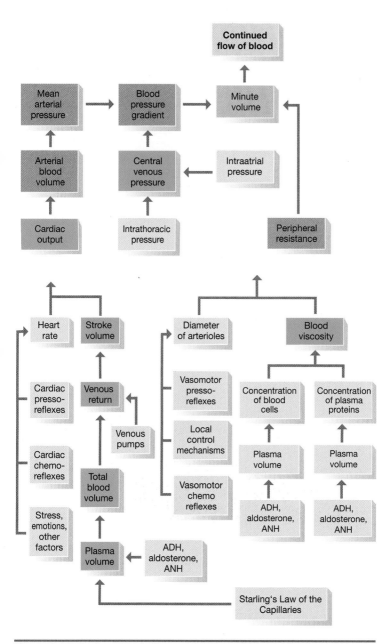

Figure 4-13 Factors that influence the flow of blood. The flow of blood, expressed as volume of blood flowing per minute (or *minute volume*), is determined by various factors. This chart shows only some of the major factors that influence blood flow. Notice that some factors appear more than once in the chart, indicating that they can influence blood flow in several ways.

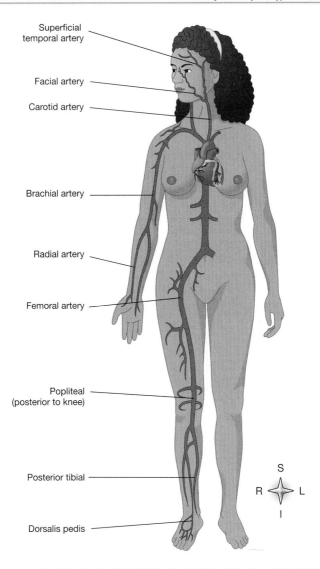

Superficial
temporal artery

Facial artery

Carotid artery

Brachial artery

Radial artery

Femoral artery

Popliteal
(posterior to knee)

Posterior tibial

Dorsalis pedis

S

R ✦ L

I

Figure 4-14 Pulse points. The pulse can be felt wherever an artery lies near the surface and over a bone or other firm background. Some of the specific locations where the pulse point is most easily felt are shown. Each pulse point is named after the artery with which it's associated.

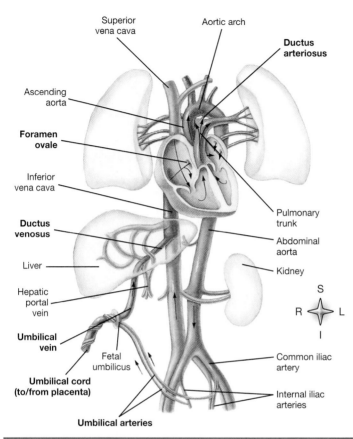

Figure 4-15 Plan of fetal circulation. Before birth, the human circulatory system has several special features that adapt the body to life in the womb. These features *(labeled in **bold** type)* include two umbilical arteries, one umbilical vein, ductus venosus, foramen ovale, ductus arteriosus, and umbilical cord. The placenta, another essential feature of the fetal circulatory plan, is not shown.

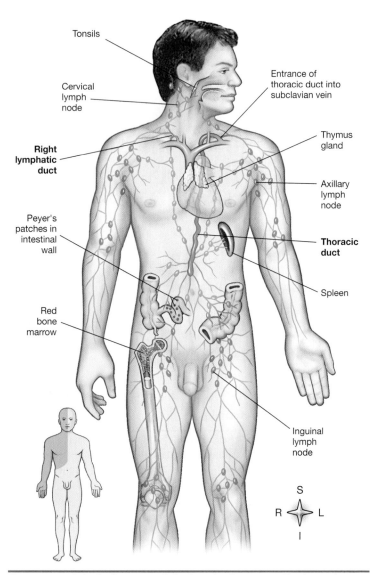

Tonsils

Cervical lymph node

Right lymphatic duct

Peyer's patches in intestinal wall

Red bone marrow

Entrance of thoracic duct into subclavian vein

Thymus gland

Axillary lymph node

Thoracic duct

Spleen

Inguinal lymph node

S

R ✦ L

I

Figure 4-16 **Principal organs of the lymphatic system.** The inset shows the areas drained by the right lymphatic duct(s) in green and the areas drained by the thoracic duct in blue.

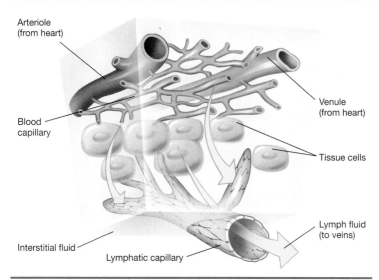

Figure 4-17 Role of the lymphatic system in fluid balance. Fluid from plasma flowing through the capillaries moves into interstitial spaces. Although *most* of this interstitial fluid (IF) is either absorbed by tissue cells or reabsorbed by capillaries, *some* of the fluid tends to accumulate in the interstitial spaces. As this fluid builds up, it tends to drain into lymphatic vessels that eventually return the fluid to the venous blood.

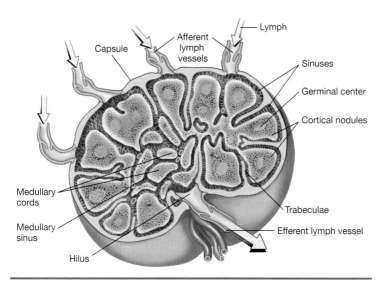

Figure 4-18 Structure of a lymph node. Several afferent-valved lymphatics bring lymph to the node. In this example, a single efferent lymphatic leaves the node at a concave area called the *hilum.* Note that the artery and vein also enter and leave at the hilum. *Arrows* show direction of lymph.

Field Notes

Sewers and Drains

The overall role of the lymphatic system in the body is always a little confusing for beginning students. Perhaps because we don't hear much about it in our culture, the way we do with nearly all the other parts of the body.

It really is pretty easy, however. The best way to understand the role of the lymphatic system is to use the analogy of the system of storm drains and sewage treatment in a city.

Let's start with the city. It rains, and the rain soaks into the ground, evaporates, or runs off into the local rivers and streams. Then the water proceeds through the water cycle. Remember the water cycle from middle school science class? That's the idea that water all eventually gets back into the clouds and returns as rain.

However, some of the rain falls on the streets, roofs, and parking lots and doesn't soak into the ground and doesn't all evaporate. Instead it runs off into drains and sewers scattered around the city. If you didn't have such drainage networks, any good rain would flood streets and homes and make a big mess all around.

Where does all that drained water go? It goes through a network of drainpipes that conduct the wastewater off toward the sewage treatment plants. Some cities don't send all wastewater to a treatment plant—but they should. At the wastewater treatment plant, the chunks of stuff that have been carried along by the storm runoff are filtered out (mechanical, or primary, filtration), and bacteria convert chemical wastes to something harmless (biological, or secondary, filtration).

Then the cleaned up wastewater goes out of the treatment plant and into the local river or lake. Now it's back in the water cycle and will someday return as rain.

Likewise, the tissues of the body are constantly being rained on by fluids that are leaving the blood capillaries. That water becomes interstitial fluid (IF); some of it is used by cells, and some of it diffuses or filters back into the bloodstream. However, some of it collects in drains—the lymphatic capillaries. This prevents "flooding" or swelling (edema) of tissues. Once in the lymphatic system, the runoff IF is called *lymph*.

The lymph collects with larger lymphatic vessels (like larger drainpipes) and goes to small little wastewater treatment plants called *lymph nodes*. As it passes through a lymph node, the lymph is mechanically and biologically filtered. Thus the lymph leaving the

Field Notes—cont'd

lymph node is relatively free of damaged cells or cell parts, bacteria, cancer cells, and so on. The cleaned up lymph then moves into larger and larger lymphatic vessels until it is eventually dumped into the bloodstream (a subclavian vein).

Thus the fluid that started out as blood plasma, then became IF, then became lymph, is now returned to the bloodstream again. The lymphatic system completes the body's form of a "water cycle" in a way that not only constantly recycles water but also prevents swelling of tissues.

Table 4-7	Mechanisms of Nonspecific Defense (Innate Immunity)

MECHANISM	DESCRIPTION
Species resistance	Genetic characteristics of human species protect the body from certain pathogens
Mechanical and chemical barriers	Physical impediments to the entry of foreign cells or substances
Skin and mucosa	Forms a continuous wall that separates the internal environment from the external environment, preventing the entry of pathogens
Secretions	Secretions such as sebum, mucus, and enzymes chemically inhibit the activity of pathogens
Inflammation	The inflammatory response isolates the pathogens and stimulates the speedy arrival of large of numbers immune cells
Phagocytosis	Ingestion and destruction of pathogens by phagocytic cells
Neutrophils	Granular leukocytes that are usually the first phagocytic cell to arrive at the scene of an inflammatory response
Macrophages	Monocytes that have enlarged to become giant phagocytic cells capable of consuming many pathogens; often called by other, more specific names when found in specific tissues of the body
Natural killer (NK) cells	Group of lymphocytes that kill many different types of cancer cells and virus-infected cells

Continued

Table 4-7	Mechanisms of Nonspecific Defense (Innate Immunity)—cont'd

MECHANISM	DESCRIPTION
Interferon	Protein produced by cells after they become infected by a virus; inhibits the spread or further development of a viral infection
Complement	Group of plasma proteins (inactive enzymes) that produce a cascade of chemical reactions that ultimately causes lysis (rupture) of a foreign cell; the complement cascade can be triggered by specific or nonspecific immune mechanisms

Foreign invaders: The body is constantly being bombarded by invading organisms, such as viruses, bacteria, and other microorganisms

1. Scavenger cells such as neutrophils arrive early at the site of invasion, but survive only a few days

2. The complement system's circulating proteins attach to microbial invaders, leading to their destruction

3. Macrophages engulf foreign matter and signal other immune cells to attack invaders

4. Macrophages display antigens from ingested invaders. These activate helper T cells

Helper T cells

5. Helper T cells multiply and activate B cells and macrophages

6. B cells divide and form plasma cells, which produce antibodies

B cell

7. Antibodies bind to invaders, either destroying them or making them more vulnerable to macrophages

8. Killer T cells form and destroy foreign invaders

9. Suppressor T cells slow or stop the immune response once the foreign invader is defeated

10. Some B and T cells become memory cells, which can quickly mount a defense if the same foreign invader attacks again

Figure 4-19 **Biologic warfare.** A brief summary of the immune response.

CHAPTER FIVE

Respiration, Nutrition, and Excretion

TOPICS

Respiratory system, digestive system, nutrition, urinary system, acid-base balance, fluid/electrolyte balance

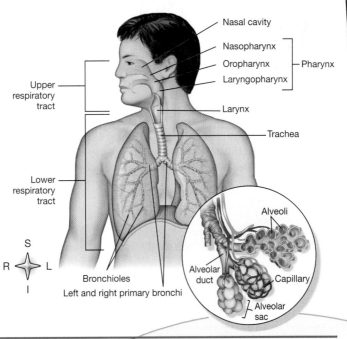

Nasal cavity

Nasopharynx
Oropharynx ⎤
Laryngopharynx ⎦ Pharynx

Upper respiratory tract

Larynx

Trachea

Lower respiratory tract

Alveoli

S
R ✛ L
I

Bronchioles
Left and right primary bronchi

Alveolar duct
Capillary

Alveolar sac

Figure 5-1 Structural plan of the respiratory system. The inset shows the alveolar sacs where the interchange of oxygen (O_2) and carbon dioxide (CO_2) takes place through the walls of the grapelike alveoli.

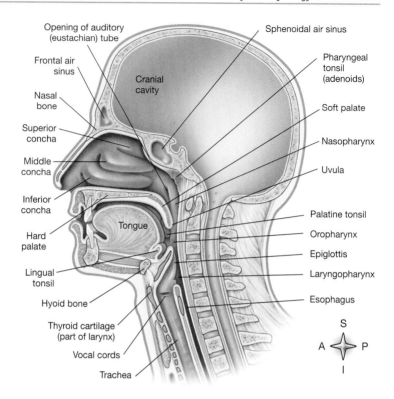

Figure 5-2 Sagittal section of the head and neck. Upper respiratory structures are clearly visible. In section through the nose and nasal cavity, the nasal septum has been removed to reveal the turbinates (nasal conchae) of the lateral wall of the nasal cavity.

Table 5-1	Pulmonary Volumes and Capacities

VOLUME	DESCRIPTION
Tidal volume (TV)	Volume moved into or out of the respiratory tract during a normal respiratory cycle
Inspiratory reserve volume (IRV)	Maximum volume that can be moved into the respiratory tract after a normal inspiration
Expiratory reserve volume (ERV)	Maximum volume that can be moved out of the respiratory tract after a normal expiration
Residual volume (RV)	Volume remaining in the respiratory tract after maximum expiration

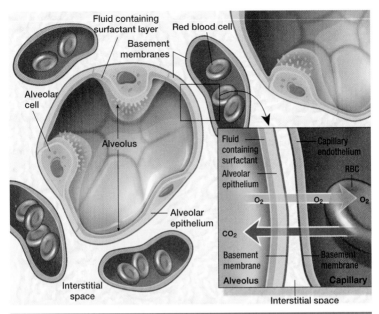

Figure 5-3 The gas exchange structures of the lung. Each alveolus is continually ventilated with fresh air. The inset shows a magnified view of the respiratory membrane composed of the alveolar wall (fluid coating, epithelial cells, and basement membrane), interstitial fluid (IF), and the wall of a pulmonary capillary (basement membrane and endothelial cells). The gases, carbon dioxide (CO_2) and oxygen (O_2), diffuse across the respiratory membrane.

TYPICAL VALUE	CAPACITY	FORMULA	TYPICAL VALUE
500 ml	Vital capacity (VC)	TV + IRV + ERV	4500-5000 ml
3000-3300 ml	Inspiratory capacity (IC)	TV + IRV	3500-3800 ml
1000-1200 ml	Functional residual capacity (FRC)	ERV + RV	2200-2400 ml
1200 ml	Total lung capacity (TLC)	TV + IRV + ERV + RV	5700-6200 ml

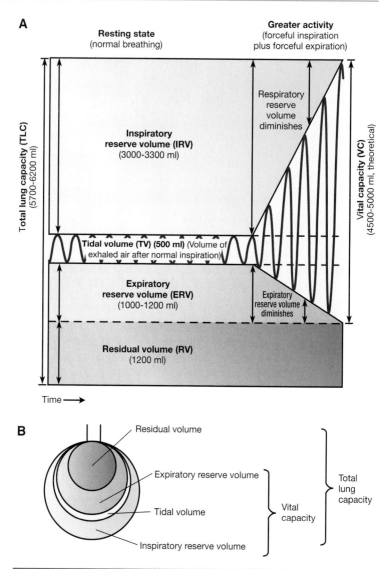

Figure 5-4 Pulmonary ventilation volumes. A, Graph produced by a spirometer. **B,** Figure showing the pulmonary volumes at rest as relative proportions of an inflated balloon. During normal, quiet respirations, the atmosphere and lungs exchange about 500 ml of air (tidal volume [TV]). With a forcible inspiration, about 3300 ml more air can be inhaled (inspiratory reserve volume [IRV]). After a normal inspiration and normal expiration, approximately 1000 ml more air can be forcibly expired (expiratory reserve volume [ERV]). Vital capacity is the amount of air that can be forcibly expired after a maximal inspiration and therefore indicates the largest amount of air that can enter and leave the lungs during respiration. Residual volume is the air that remains trapped in the alveoli.

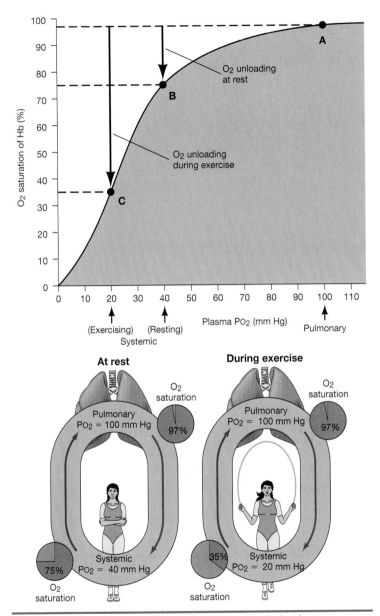

Figure 5-5 **Oxyhemoglobin dissociation curve.** Graph showing oxygen (O_2) unloading at rest and during exercise. At rest, fully saturated hemoglobin (Hb) unloads almost 25% of its O_2 load when it reaches the low O_2 partial pressure (PO_2) (40 mm Hg) environment in systemic tissues *(left)*. During exercise, the tissue PO_2 is even lower (20 mm Hg)—thus causing fully saturated Hb to unload about 70% of its O_2 load *(right)*. As you can see in the graph, a slight drop in tissue PO_2—from point *B* to point *C*—causes a large increase in O_2 unloading *(top)*.

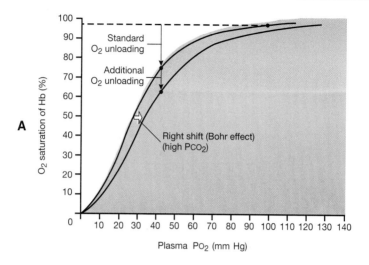

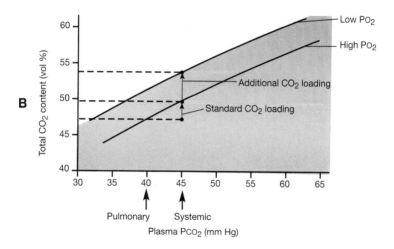

Figure 5-6 Interaction of oxygen partial pressure and carbon dioxide partial pressure on gas transport by the blood. A, The increased carbon dioxide partial pressure (Pco$_2$) in systemic tissues decreases the affinity between hemoglobin (Hb) and oxygen (O$_2$), shown as a right shift of the O$_2$-Hb dissociation curve. This phenomenon is known as the *Bohr effect*. A right shift can also be caused by a decrease in plasma pH. **B,** At the same time, the decreased oxygen partial pressure (Po$_2$) commonly observed in systemic tissues increases the carbon dioxide (CO$_2$) content of the blood, shown as a left shift of the CO$_2$ dissociation curve. This phenomenon is known as the *Haldane effect*.

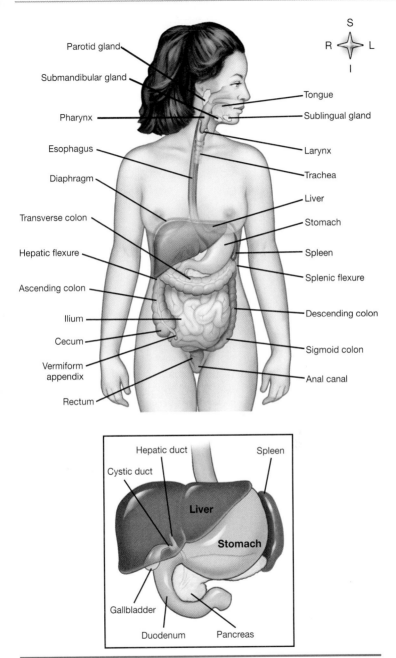

Figure 5-7 Location of digestive organs. Inset shows a closer view of the upper abdominal organs. A few nondigestive organs are shown to clarify positions in the body.

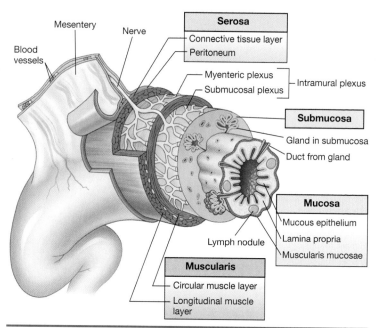

Figure 5-8 Wall of the gastrointestinal tract. The wall of the gastrointestinal (GI) tract is made up of four layers, shown here in a generalized diagram of a segment of the GI tract. Notice that the serosa is continuous with a fold of serous membrane called a mesentery. Notice also that digestive glands may empty their products into the lumen of the GI tract by way of ducts.

Table 5-2	Modifications of Layers of the Digestive Tract Wall		
ORGAN	MUCOSA	MUSCULARIS	SEROSA
Esophagus	Stratified squamous epithelium resists abrasion	Two layers—inner one of circular fibers and outer one of longitudinal fibers; striated muscle in upper part and smooth muscle in lower part of esophagus and in rest of tract	Outer layer fibrous (adventitia); serous around part of esophagus in thoracic cavity

Table 5-2	Modifications of Layers of the Digestive Tract Wall—cont'd		
ORGAN	**MUCOSA**	**MUSCULARIS**	**SEROSA**
Stomach	Arranged in flexible longitudinal folds, called *rugae*; allow for distention; contains gastric pits with microscopic gastric glands	Has three layers instead of usual two —circular, longitudinal, and oblique fibers; two sphincters—lower esophageal at entrance of stomach and pyloric at its exit, formed by circular fibers	Outer layer, visceral peritoneum; hangs in double fold from lower edge of stomach over intestines, forming apronlike structure; greater omentum; lesser omentum connects stomach to liver
Small intestine	Contains permanent circular folds, plicae circulares	Two layers—inner one of circular fibers and outer one of longitudinal fibers	Outer layer, visceral peritoneum, continuous with mesentery
	Microscopic fingerlike projections, villi with brush border		
	Crypts (of Lieberkühn)		
	Microscopic duodenal (Brunner) mucous glands		
	Clusters of lymph nodules (Peyer's patches)		
	Numerous single lymph nodes, called *solitary nodes*		

Continued

Table 5-2   Modifications of Layers of the Digestive Tract Wall—cont'd

ORGAN	MUCOSA	MUSCULARIS	SEROSA
Large intestine	Solitary lymph nodes	Outer longitudinal layer condensed to form three tapelike strips *(taeniae coli);* small sacs (haustra) give rest of wall of large intestine puckered appearance; internal anal sphincter formed by circular smooth fibers; external anal sphincter formed by striated fibers	Outer layer, visceral peritoneum, continuous with mesocolon
	Intestinal mucous glands		
	Anal columns form in anal region		

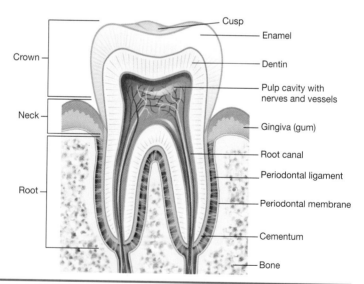

Figure 5-9 Typical tooth. Molar tooth sectioned to show its bony socket and details of its three main parts: crown, neck, and root. Enamel *(over the crown)* and cementum *(over the neck and root)* surround the dentin layer. The pulp contains nerves and blood vessels.

Table 5-3 Dentition

NAME OF TOOTH	NUMBER PER JAW	
	DECIDUOUS SET	PERMANENT SET
Central incisors	2	2
Lateral incisors	2	2
Canines (cuspids)	2	2
Premolars (bicuspids)	0	4
First molars (tricuspids)	2	2
Second molars	2	2
Third molars (wisdom teeth)	0	2
Total (Per Jaw)	10	16
Total (Per Set)	20	32

Field Notes

Swiss Army Knife

Despite being officially neutral, the Swiss have gained a reputation for excellence in military technology and training. It is no wonder that the famous "Swiss army knife" concept has been adopted by so many around the world for so many different uses.

The idea of a Swiss military knife is that it is basically a regular, folding pocket knife but with many extra gadgets. Besides a knife, it usually contains several different tiny screwdrivers, a very small can opener, a miniature corkscrew (I guess the Swiss army is rationed very small bottles of Swiss wine with tiny corks), a tiny saw blade, and several other really tiny implements. These knifes are great because they are easy to carry around (except into secure buildings) but have the capability of a wide assortment of different tools. It's like having a whole tool set in your pocket. This idea has become so popular that now you can get versions with all kinds of different things in them, such as laser pointers and other modern gadgets.

The drawback with this style of knife is that to make it "handy," all the little tools are really tiny. The itty-bitty screwdriver is great for an emergency repair—but you wouldn't want to put together your new "needs some assembly" furniture with it. That little corkscrew is cool, but would a wine steward really use one of those? Nope. In other words, each one of those tools is great for an occasional use while "traveling light" but does not have the full capability of the larger, independent version of the tool.

Continued

Field Notes—cont'd

This is analogous to the dentition of the human mouth. Dentition is the kind and numbers of teeth in an organism.

Human dentition is outlined in Figure 5-10 and listed in Table 5-3. Humans are classified as omnivores, meaning that we have the ability to eat and digest a wide variety of different organisms: plants, animals, fungi, and more. Herbivores have a different sort of dentition because they mainly eat plants. Therefore herbivores, like horses and rabbits, have really big incisors for biting off plants and really broad, flat molars for grinding it up. Carnivores have the sort of dentition needed for eating mainly animals. Carnivores, like cats and dogs, have really small incisors but really big, pointed canines for killing animals and tearing meat. Their premolars and molars are like saw blades for cutting through meat and bone.

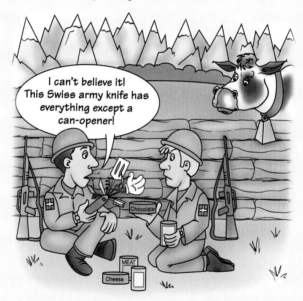

Humans, being omnivores, have a sort of *Swiss army knife dentition*. That is, we have one of everything that both the herbivores and carnivores have, but none of ours are very capable in comparison. For example, our incisors can bite off a carrot but not a tree limb. Our canines can help rip the meat from barbeque ribs but not the thigh muscles from an antelope. Our molars can grind up some salad but not raw whole oats—at least not very effectively. Therefore our mouth has a variety of moderately useful tools. This analogy also helps us understand the role of teeth: they are tools. Think about how you use the different types of teeth in your mouth (for biting and chewing).

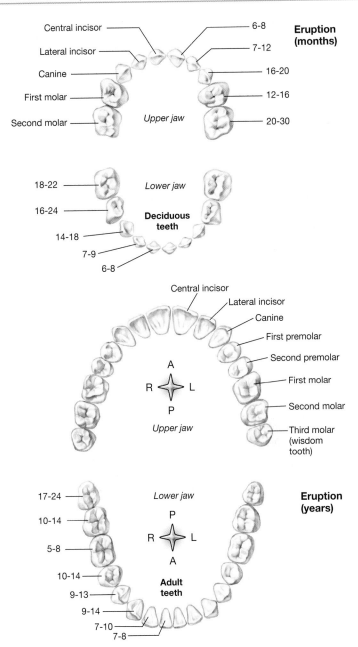

Figure 5-10 Dentition. Deciduous (baby) teeth and adult teeth are shown. No premolars exist in the deciduous set, and only two pairs of molars are found in each jaw. Generally the lower teeth erupt before the corresponding upper teeth.

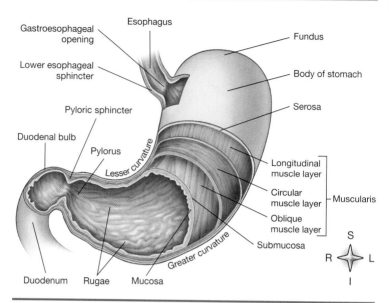

Figure 5-11 Stomach. A portion of the anterior wall has been cut away to reveal the muscle layers of the stomach wall. Notice that the mucosa lining the stomach forms folds called *rugae*.

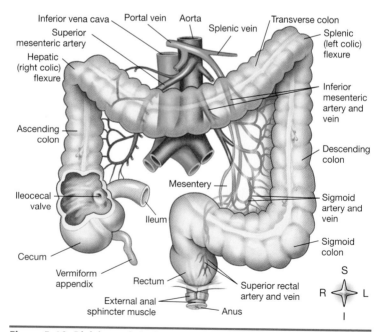

Figure 5-12 Divisions of the large intestine. Illustration showing divisions of the large intestine and adjacent vascular structures.

Table 5-4	Primary Mechanisms of the Digestive System

MECHANISM	DESCRIPTION
Ingestion	Process of taking food into the mouth, starting it on its journey through the digestive tract
Digestion	A group of processes that break complex nutrients into simpler ones, thus facilitating their absorption; *mechanical digestion* physically breaks large chunks into small bits; *chemical digestion* breaks molecules apart
Motility	Movement by the muscular components of the digestive tube, including processes of mechanical digestion; examples include *peristalsis* and *segmentation*
Secretion	Release of digestive juices (containing enzymes, acids, bases, mucus, bile, or other products that facilitate digestion); some digestive organs also secrete endocrine hormones that regulate digestion or metabolism of nutrients
Absorption	Movement of digested nutrients through the gastrointestinal (GI) mucosa and into the internal environment
Elimination	Excretion of the residues of the digestive process (feces) from the rectum, through the anus; defecation

Table 5-5	Processes of Mechanical Digestion	

ORGAN	MECHANICAL PROCESS	NATURE OF PROCESS
Mouth (teeth and tongue)	Mastication	Chewing movements (reduce size of food particles and mix them with saliva)
	Deglutition	Swallowing (movement of food from mouth to stomach)
Pharynx	Deglutition	
Esophagus	Deglutition	
	Peristalsis	Rippling movements that squeeze food downward in digestive tract; constricted ring forms first in one section and then the next, causing waves of contraction to spread along entire canal
Stomach	Churning	Forward and backward movement of gastric contents, mixing food with gastric juices to form chyme
	Peristalsis	Wave starting in body of stomach about three times per minute and sweeping toward closed pyloric sphincter; at intervals, strong peristaltic waves press chyme past sphincter into duodenum

Continued

Table 5-5 Processes of Mechanical Digestion—cont'd

ORGAN	MECHANICAL PROCESS	NATURE OF PROCESS
Small Intestine		
	Segmentation (mixing contractions) Peristalsis	Forward and backward movement within segment of intestine; purpose is to mix food and digestive juices thoroughly and to bring all digested food in contact with intestinal mucosa to facilitate absorption; purpose of peristalsis, on the other hand, is to propel intestinal contents along digestive tract
Large Intestine		
Colon	Segmentation Peristalsis	Churning movements within haustral sacs
Descending colon	Mass peristalsis	Entire contents moved into sigmoid colon and rectum; occurs three or four times a day, usually after a meal
Rectum	Defecation	Emptying of rectum, so-called bowel movement

Table 5-6 Chemical Digestion

DIGESTIVE JUICES AND ENZYMES	SUBSTANCE DIGESTED (OR HYDROLYZED)	RESULTING PRODUCT*
Saliva		
Amylase	Starch (polysaccharide)	Maltose (a double sugar, or disaccharide)
Gastric Juice		
Protease (pepsin) plus hydrochloric acid	Proteins	Partially digested
Pancreatic Juice		
Proteases (e.g., trypsin)†	Proteins (intact or partially digested)	Peptides and **amino acids**

*Substances in **boldface type** are end-products of digestion (that is, completely digested nutrients ready for absorption).

†Secreted in inactive form (trypsinogen); activated by enterokinase, an enzyme in the intestinal brush border.

‡Brush-border enzymes.

§Glucose is also called *dextrose*; fructose is also called *levulose*.

Table 5-6   Chemical Digestion—cont'd

DIGESTIVE JUICES AND ENZYMES	SUBSTANCE DIGESTED (OR HYDROLYZED)	RESULTING PRODUCT*
Lipases	Fats emulsified by bile	**Fatty acids, monoglycerides, and glycerol**
Intestinal Enzymes‡		
Peptidases	Peptides	Amino acids
Sucrase	Sucrose (cane sugar)	**Glucose and fructose§** (simple sugars or monosaccharides)
Lactase	Lactose (milk sugar)	**Glucose and galactose** (simple sugars)
Maltase	Maltose (malt sugar)	**Glucose**

Table 5-7   Digestive Secretions

DIGESTIVE JUICE	SOURCE	SUBSTANCE	FUNCTIONAL ROLE*
Saliva	Salivary glands	Mucus	*Lubricates bolus of food; facilitates mixing of food*
		Amylase	**Enzyme; begins digestion of starches**
		Sodium bicarbonate	Increases pH (for optimum amylase function)
		Water	*Dilutes food and other substances; facilitates mixing*
Gastric juice	Gastric glands	Pepsin	**Enzyme; digests proteins**
		Hydrochloric acid	**Denatures proteins; decreases pH (for optimum pepsin function)**
		Intrinsic factor	**Protects and allows later absorption of vitamin B_{12}**
		Mucus	*Lubricates chyme; protects stomach lining*
		Water	*Dilutes food and other substances; facilitates mixing*

Continued

Table 5-7 Digestive Secretions—cont'd

DIGESTIVE JUICE	SOURCE	SUBSTANCE	FUNCTIONAL ROLE*
Pancreatic juice	Pancreas (exocrine portion)	Proteases (trypsin, chymotrypsin, collagenase, elastase)	**Enzymes; digest proteins and polypeptides**
		Lipases (lipase, phospholipase)	**Enzymes; digest lipids**
		Colipase	**Coenzyme; helps lipase digest fats**
		Nucleases	**Enzymes; digest nucleic acids (RNA and DNA)**
		Amylase	**Enzyme; digests starches**
		Water	*Dilutes food and other substances; facilitates mixing*
		Mucus	*Lubricates*
		Sodium bicarbonate	**Increases pH (for optimum enzyme function)**
Bile	Liver (stored and concentrated in gallbladder)	Lecithin and bile salts	*Emulsify lipids*
		Sodium bicarbonate	**Increases pH (for optimum enzyme function)**
		Cholesterol	Excess cholesterol from body cells, to be excreted with feces
		Products of detoxification	From detoxification of harmful substances by hepatic cells, to be excreted with feces
		Bile pigments (mainly bilirubin)	Products of breakdown of heme groups during hemolysis, to be excreted with feces
		Mucus	*Lubrication*
		Water	*Dilutes food and other substances; facilitates mixing*
Intestinal juice	Mucosa of small and large intestine	Mucus	*Lubrication*
		Sodium bicarbonate	**Increases pH (for optimum enzyme function)**
		Water	*Small amount to carry mucus and sodium bicarbonate*

***Boldface** type indicates a chemical digestive process; italic type indicates a mechanical digestive process.

Field Notes

Keep It Moving

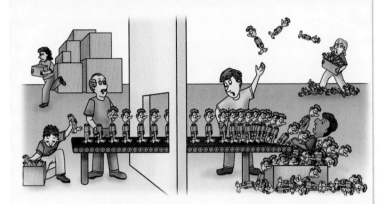

The phases of gastric secretion outlined in Figure 5-13 seem pretty complicated at first glance. However, this diagram is not only a simplification of a much more complex process than shown but also just one of many examples of regulation in the whole digestive tract.

What advantage is all this complexity? The short answer is that it helps us keep things moving along in a coordinated way. Without such coordination, your midday meal might be whisked along from the stomach to the small intestine before room exists to receive it. In addition, when the meal does begin moving from the stomach, you don't want it to all move at once—the intestines are too narrow to handle it. You also need to make sure that digestive juices are being released into the intestines at the same time as the meal is entering—otherwise it won't be digested properly.

The analogy of a factory assembly line is a good one for understanding digestive regulation. A number of nervous, hormonal, and local regulatory mechanisms make sure that one part of your "food processing line" is not going faster than the part that comes next. In addition, these mechanisms make sure that each process has the secretions it needs to be effective, the motility (muscle activity) needed to move things along or swish them around a little, and the proper pH for the enzymes to do their jobs.

Think of this analogy as you review Figure 5-13 and Table 5-8.

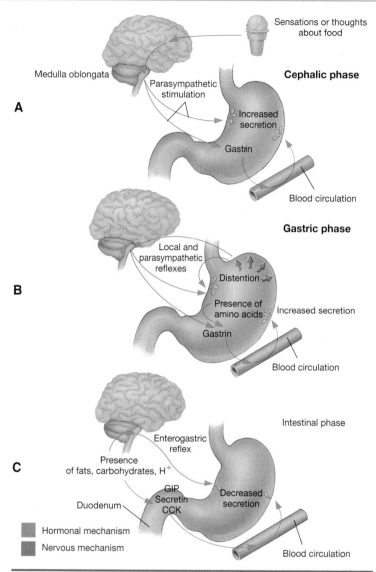

Figure 5-13 **Phases of gastric secretion. A, Cephalic phase.** Sensations of thoughts about food are relayed to the brainstem, where parasympathetic signals to the gastric mucosa are initiated. This directly stimulates gastric juice secretion and also stimulates the release of gastrin, which prolongs and enhances the effect. **B, Gastric phase.** The presence of food, specifically the distention it causes, triggers local and parasympathetic nervous reflexes that increase secretion of gastric juice and gastrin (which further amplifies gastric juice secretion). Products of protein digestion can also trigger the gastrin mechanism. **C, Intestinal phase.** As food moves into the duodenum, the presence of fats, carbohydrates, and acid stimulate hormonal and nervous reflexes that inhibit stomach activity.

Table 5-8	Actions of Some Digestive Hormones Summarized	
HORMONE	**SOURCE**	**ACTION**
Gastrin	Formed by gastric mucosa in presence of partially digested proteins, when stimulated by the vagus nerve, or when the stomach is stretched	Stimulate secretion of gastric juice rich in pepsin and hydrochloric acid
Gastric inhibitory peptide	Formed by intestinal mucosa in presence of fats and perhaps other nutrients	Inhibits gastric secretion and motility
Secretin	Formed by intestinal mucosa in presence of acid, partially digested proteins, and fats	Inhibits gastric secretion; stimulates secretion of pancreatic juice low in enzymes and high in alkalinity (bicarbonate); stimulates ejection of bile by the gallbladder
Cholecystokinin (CCK)	Formed by intestinal mucosa in presence of fats, partially digested proteins, and acids	Stimulates ejection of bile from gallbladder and secretion of pancreatic juice high in enzymes; opposes the action of gastrin, raising the pH of gastric juice

Table 5-9	Food Absorption	
FORM ABSORBED	**STRUCTURES INTO WHICH ABSORBED**	**CIRCULATION**
Protein (as amino acids) Perhaps minute quantities of some short-chain polypeptides and whole proteins absorbed (e.g., some antibodies)	Blood in intestinal capillaries	Portal vein, liver, hepatic vein, inferior vena cava to heart

Continued

Table 5-9 Food Absorption—cont'd

FORM ABSORBED	STRUCTURES INTO WHICH ABSORBED	CIRCULATION
Carbohydrates (as simple sugars)	Same as amino acids	Same as amino acids
Fats		
Glycerol and monoglycerides	Lymph in intestinal lacteals	During absorption, that is, while in epithelial cells of intestinal mucosa, glycerol and fatty acids recombine to form microscopic packages of fats (chylomicrons); lymphatics carry them by way of thoracic duct to left subclavian vein, superior vena cava, heart; some fats transported by blood in form of phospholipids or cholesterol esters
Fatty acids combine with bile salts to form water-soluble substance	Lymph in intestinal lacteals	
Some finely emulsified, undigested fats absorbed	Small fraction enters intestinal blood capillaries	

Table 5-10 Amino Acids

ESSENTIAL (INDISPENSABLE)	NONESSENTIAL (DISPENSABLE)
Histidine*	Alanine
Isoleucine	Arginine
Leucine	Asparagine
Lysine	Aspartic acid
Methionine	Cysteine
Phenylalanine	Glutamic acid
Threonine	Glutamine
Tryptophan	Glycine
Valine	Proline
	Serine
	Tyrosine†

*Essential in infants and, perhaps, adult men.

†Can be synthesized from phenylalanine; therefore is nonessential as long as phenylalanine is in the diet.

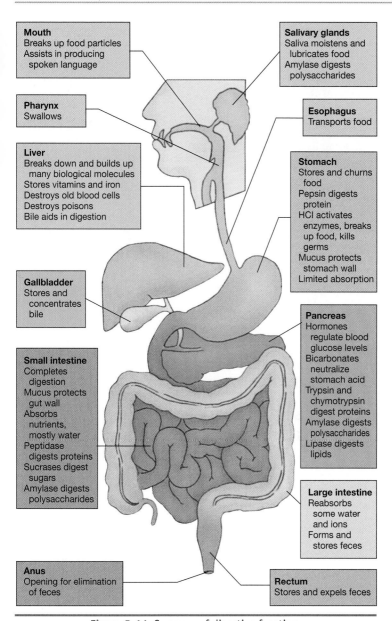

Mouth
Breaks up food particles
Assists in producing
spoken language

Salivary glands
Saliva moistens and
lubricates food
Amylase digests
polysaccharides

Pharynx
Swallows

Esophagus
Transports food

Liver
Breaks down and builds up
many biological molecules
Stores vitamins and iron
Destroys old blood cells
Destroys poisons
Bile aids in digestion

Stomach
Stores and churns
food
Pepsin digests
protein
HCl activates
enzymes, breaks
up food, kills
germs
Mucus protects
stomach wall
Limited absorption

Gallbladder
Stores and
concentrates
bile

Pancreas
Hormones
regulate blood
glucose levels
Bicarbonates
neutralize
stomach acid
Trypsin and
chymotrypsin
digest proteins
Amylase digests
polysaccharides
Lipase digests
lipids

Small intestine
Completes
digestion
Mucus protects
gut wall
Absorbs
nutrients,
mostly water
Peptidase
digests proteins
Sucrases digest
sugars
Amylase digests
polysaccharides

Large intestine
Reabsorbs
some water
and ions
Forms and
stores feces

Anus
Opening for elimination
of feces

Rectum
Stores and expels feces

Figure 5-14 Summary of digestive function.

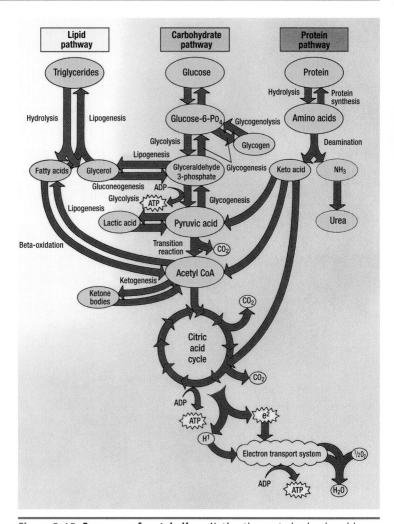

Figure 5-15 Summary of metabolism. Notice the central role played by the citric acid cycle and electron transport system. Notice also how different nutrient molecules can be converted to forms that may enter other pathways.

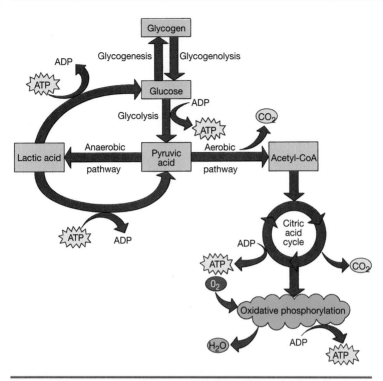

Figure 5-16 Summary of glucose metabolism. Glucose is catabolized to pyruvic acid in the process of glycolysis. If oxygen (O_2) is available, pyruvic acid is converted to acetyl coenzyme A (acetyl-CoA) and then enters the citric acid cycle and transfers energy to the maximum number of adenosine triphosphate (ATP) molecules via oxidative phosphorylation. If O_2 is not available, pyruvic acid is converted to lactic acid, incurring an O_2 debt. The O_2 debt is later repaid when ATP produced via oxidative phosphorylation is used to convert lactic acid back into pyruvic acid or all the way back to glucose. If an excess of glucose exists, the cell may convert it to glycogen (glycogenesis). Later individual glucose molecules can be removed from the glycogen chain by the process of glycogenolysis. Although nicotinamide-adenine dinucleotide (NAD) and flavin adenine dinucleotide (FAD) play important roles in these pathways, they have been left out of this diagram for the sake of simplicity.

Table 5-11 Metabolism

NUTRIENT	ANABOLISM	CATABOLISM
Carbohydrates	Temporary excess changed into glycogen by liver cells in presence of insulin; stored in liver and skeletal muscles until needed and then changed back to glucose	Oxidized, in presence of insulin, to yield energy (4.1 kcal/g) and wastes (carbon dioxide [CO_2] and water [H_2O])
	True excess beyond body's energy requirements converted into adipose tissue; stored in various fat depots of body	$C_6H_{12}O_6 + 6\ O_2 \rightarrow$ Energy + $6\ CO_2 + 6\ H_2O$
Fats	Built into adipose tissue; stored in fat depots of body	Fatty acids $\downarrow$ (beta-oxidation) Acetyl CoA $\rightleftarrows$ Ketones $\downarrow$ (tissues, citric acid cycle) Energy (9.3 kcal/g) + CO_2 + and H_2O Glycerol $\downarrow$ (glycolysis) Acetyl-CoA
Proteins	Synthesized into tissue proteins, blood proteins, enzymes, hormones, etc.	Deaminated by liver, forming ammonia (which is converted to urea) and keto acids (which are either oxidized or changed to glucose or fat)

Table 5-12 Major Vitamins

VITAMIN	DIETARY SOURCE	FUNCTIONS	SYMPTOMS OF DEFICIENCY
Vitamin A	Green and yellow vegetables, dairy products, and liver	Maintains epithelial tissue and produces visual pigments	Night blindness and flaking skin
B-Complex Vitamins			
B_1 (thiamine)	Grains, meat, and legumes	Helps enzymes in the citric acid cycle	Nerve problems (beriberi), heart muscle weakness, and edema

Table 5-12   Major Vitamins—cont'd

VITAMIN	DIETARY SOURCE	FUNCTIONS	SYMPTOMS OF DEFICIENCY
B_2 (riboflavin)	Green vegetables, organ meats, eggs, and dairy products	Aids enzymes in the citric acid cycle	Inflammation of skin and eyes
B_3 (niacin)	Meat and grains	Helps enzymes in the citric acid cycle	Pellagra (scaly dermatitis and mental disturbances) and nervous disorders
B_5 (pantothenic acid)	Organ meat, eggs, and liver	Aids enzymes that connect fat and carbohydrate metabolism	Loss of coordination (rare)
B_6 (pyridoxine)	Vegetables, meats, and grains	Helps enzymes that catabolize amino acids	Convulsions, irritability, and anemia
B_9 (folic acid)	Vegetables	Aids enzymes in amino acid catabolism and blood production	Digestive disorders and anemia
B_{12} (cyanocobalamin)	Meat and dairy products	Involved in blood production and other processes	Pernicious anemia
Biotin (vitamin H)	Vegetables, meat, and eggs	Helps enzymes in amino acid catabolism and fat and glycogen synthesis	Mental and muscle problems (rare)
Vitamin C (Ascorbic Acid)	Fruits and green vegetables	Helps in manufacture of collagen fibers; antioxidant	Scurvy and degeneration of skin, bone, and blood vessels
Vitamin D (Calciferol)	Dairy products and fish liver oil	Aids in calcium absorption	Rickets and skeletal deformity
Vitamin E (Tocopherol)	Green vegetables and seeds	Protects cell membranes from being destroyed	Muscle and reproductive disorders (rare)

Table 5-13   Major Minerals

MINERAL	DIETARY SOURCE	FUNCTIONS	SYMPTOMS OF DEFICIENCY
Calcium (Ca)	Dairy products, legumes, and vegetables	Helps blood clotting, bone formation, and nerve and muscle function	Bone degeneration and nerve and muscle malfunction
Chlorine (Cl)	Salty foods	Aids in stomach acid production and acid-base balance	Acid-base imbalance
Cobalt (Co)	Meat	Helps vitamin B_{12} in blood cell production	Pernicious anemia
Copper (Cu)	Seafood, organ meats, and legumes	Involved in extracting energy from the citric acid cycle and in blood production	Fatigue and anemia
Iodine (I)	Seafood and iodized salt	Required for thyroid hormone synthesis	Goiter (thyroid enlargement) and decrease of metabolic rate
Iron (Fe)	Meat, eggs, vegetables, and legumes	Involved in extracting energy from the citric acid cycle and in blood production	Fatigue and anemia
Magnesium (Mg)	Vegetables and grains	Helps many enzymes	Nerve disorders, blood vessel dilation, and heart rhythm problems
Manganese (Mn)	Vegetables, legumes, and grains	Helps many enzymes	Muscle and nerve disorders
Phosphorus (P)	Dairy products and meat	Aids in bone formation and is used to make adenosine triphosphate (ATP), deoxyribonucleic acid (DNA), ribonucleic acid (RNA), and phospholipids	Bone degeneration and metabolic problems

		Table 5-13	Major Minerals—cont'd		

MINERAL	DIETARY SOURCE	FUNCTIONS	SYMI OF D
Potassium (K)	Seafood, milk, fruit, and meats	Helps muscle and nerve function	Muscle weakness, heart problems, and nerve problems
Sodium (Na)	Salty foods	Aids in muscle and nerve function and fluid balance	Weakness and digestive upset
Zinc (Zn)	Many foods	Helps many enzymes	Inadequate growth

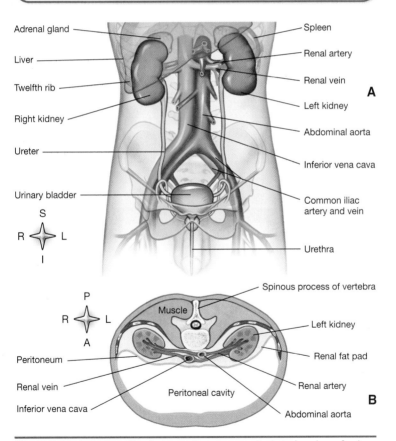

Figure 5-17 **Location of urinary system organs. A,** Anterior view of urinary organs with the peritoneum and visceral organs removed. **B,** Horizontal (transverse) section of the abdomen showing the retroperitoneal position of the kidneys.

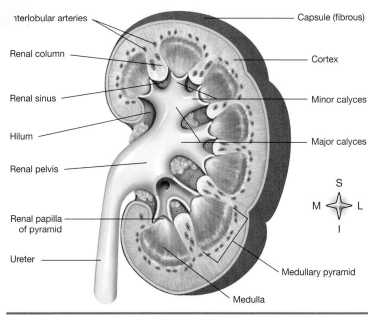

Figure 5-18 Gross structure of the kidney. Coronal section of a kidney in an artist's rendering.

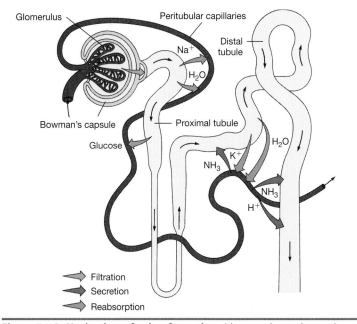

Figure 5-19 Mechanism of urine formation. Diagram shows the mechanisms of urine formation (filtration, reabsorption, and secretion) and where they occur in the nephron (microscopic functional unit of the kidney).

Field Notes

Cleaning Your Drawers

Kidney function, especially the processes within the nephrons, is often troublesome for beginning students. It needn't be, because the basic concepts are fairly simple and straightforward—once you know the overall plan. That's the tricky part. If you just dive right into it without considering the overall plan, then it doesn't seem to add up.

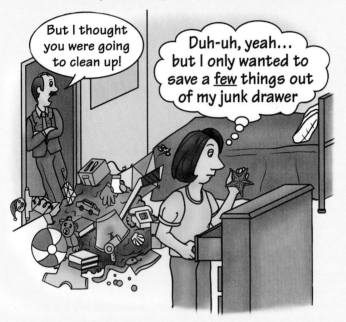

One way to think of the kidney's function is that it balances—or cleans up—the blood passing through it. Each nephron has the job of doing its small share of the cleanup duties. The three basic methods the nephron uses to do its job are outlined in Figure 5-22: filtration, reabsorption, and secretion. However, that figure looks like things are coming into and out of the blood and nothing is being "cleaned up" or balanced.

Here's an analogy that may help: You are going to clean out your junk drawer. You must be really bored—or are really trying to avoid studying. In any case you realize that your drawer contains a lot of junk and not much that is very useful. Besides, it's so packed that you probably won't be able to close it up again.

Therefore you decide that the best method would be to dump the entire contents of the drawer out onto a clear spot on the floor. That is,

Continued

Field Notes—cont'd

after you've cleared a spot on the floor. Now you can see all the stuff, all spread out. This is like filtration. When the bloodstream first hits the nephron (at the glomerulus), a huge amount of fluid and solutes moves into the Bowman's capsule. Somewhere around 50 gallons a day! Obviously, you don't want to get rid of all of it; but you dump that much into the nephron so that the nephron can decide what to keep (put back into the blood) and what not to keep (release as urine).

The next step is to pick up those things you want to keep and put them back into your junk drawer. This is like reabsorption. The cells in the wall of the nephron are constructed in a way that promotes the movement of most of the water and sodium and chloride and glucose (and a few other needed molecules) back into the blood. Recall that the bloodstream has returned again to the nephron (in the peritubular blood supply) before leaving the kidney.

Before you're done cleaning your junk drawer, you decide that some last-minute adjustments are needed. You probably should get rid of those licorice candies stuck to the side of the drawer and that old chocolate, too. Therefore you pull those off the inside of the drawer, one by one, and put them into your "trash pile" on the floor. This is like secretion. That's the process by which the nephron cells push molecules from the peritubular blood into the lumen of the nephron—where they'll be lost with the urine.

The final step, of course, is taking the trash out of your home. This is like moving the fluid in the nephron into the emptying system of the kidney: the calyces, pelvis, ureter, bladder, and urethra and then out. Once it leaves the microscopic kidney tubules, the fluid—now entirely waste—is called *urine*.

Table 5-14	Volumes of Body Fluid Compartments*		
BODY FLUID	**INFANT**	**ADULT MALE**	**ADULT FEMALE**
Extracellular Fluid (ECF)			
Plasma	4	4	4
Interstitial fluid (IF)	26	16	11
Intracellular Fluid (ICF)	45	40	35
Total	75	60	50

*Percentage of body weight.

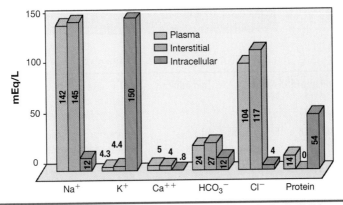

Figure 5-20 Electrolyte and protein concentrations in body fluid compartments. This illustration compares individual electrolyte and protein concentration in the three fluid compartments.

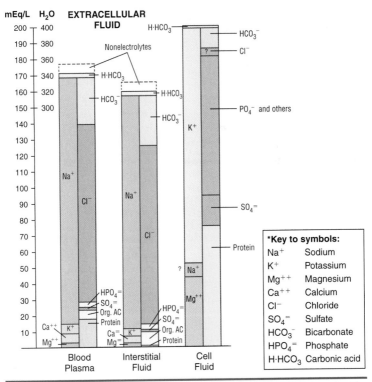

Figure 5-21 Chief chemical constituents of three fluid compartments. The column of figures at the left (e.g., 200, 190, 180) indicates amounts of cation (positive ion) or of anion (negative ion), whereas the figures on the right (e.g., 400, 380, 360) indicate the combined sum of all the cations and anions.

Table 5-15 pH Control Systems

TYPE	RESPONSE TIME	EXAMPLE
Chemical buffer systems	Immediate	Bicarbonate buffer system Phosphate buffer system Protein buffer system
Physiologic buffer systems	Minutes Hours	Respiratory response system Renal response system

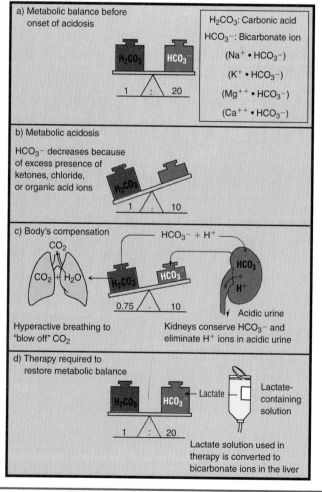

a) Metabolic balance before onset of acidosis

H_2CO_3: Carbonic acid
HCO_3^-: Bicarbonate ion
$(Na^+ \cdot HCO_3^-)$
$(K^+ \cdot HCO_3^-)$
$(Mg^{++} \cdot HCO_3^-)$
$(Ca^{++} \cdot HCO_3^-)$

H_2CO_3 HCO_3^- 1 : 20

b) Metabolic acidosis

HCO_3^- decreases because of excess presence of ketones, chloride, or organic acid ions

H_2CO_3 1 : 10

c) Body's compensation

CO_2

$HCO_3^- + H^+$

$CO_2 + H_2O$

H_2CO_3 HCO_3 0.75 : 10

HCO_3
H^+
Acidic urine

Hyperactive breathing to "blow off" CO_2

Kidneys conserve HCO_3^- and eliminate H^+ ions in acidic urine

d) Therapy required to restore metabolic balance

H_2CO_3 HCO_3 1 : 20

Lactate

Lactate-containing solution

Lactate solution used in therapy is converted to bicarbonate ions in the liver

Figure 5-22 Metabolic acidosis.

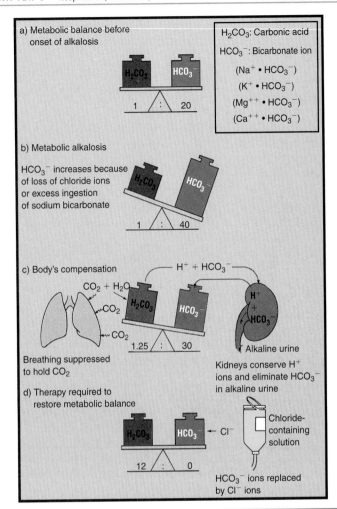

a) Metabolic balance before onset of alkalosis

H_2CO_3: Carbonic acid

HCO_3^-: Bicarbonate ion

$(Na^+ \cdot HCO_3^-)$
$(K^+ \cdot HCO_3^-)$
$(Mg^{++} \cdot HCO_3^-)$
$(Ca^{++} \cdot HCO_3^-)$

H_2CO_3 HCO_3^-

1 : 20

b) Metabolic alkalosis

HCO_3^- increases because of loss of chloride ions or excess ingestion of sodium bicarbonate

H_2CO_3 HCO_3^-

1 : 40

c) Body's compensation

$H^+ + HCO_3^-$

$CO_2 + H_2O$

CO_2
CO_2

H_2CO_3 HCO_3^-

H^+
+
HCO_3^-

1.25 : 30

Alkaline urine

Breathing suppressed to hold CO_2

Kidneys conserve H^+ ions and eliminate HCO_3^- in alkaline urine

d) Therapy required to restore metabolic balance

H_2CO_3 HCO_3^- ← Cl^-

Chloride-containing solution

12 : 0

HCO_3^- ions replaced by Cl^- ions

Figure 5-23 Metabolic alkalosis.

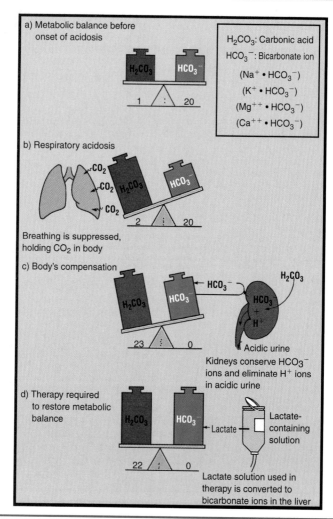

Figure 5-24 Respiratory acidosis.

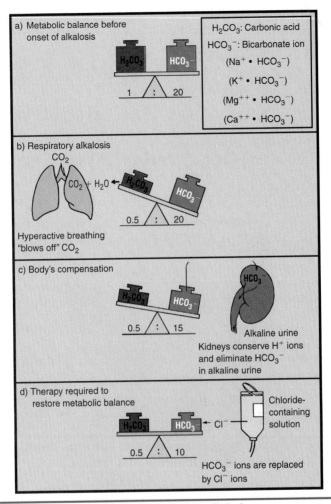

Figure 5-25 Respiratory alkalosis.

CHAPTER SIX

Reproduction and Development

TOPICS

Male reproductive system, female reproductive system, development, genetics

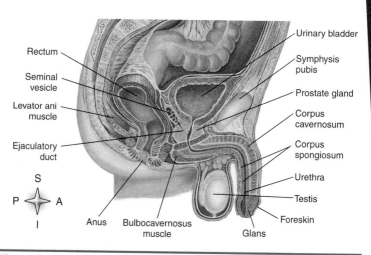

Rectum

Seminal vesicle

Levator ani muscle

Ejaculatory duct

Urinary bladder

Symphysis pubis

Prostate gland

Corpus cavernosum

Corpus spongiosum

Urethra

Testis

Foreskin

S

P — A

I

Anus

Bulbocavernosus muscle

Glans

Figure 6-1 Male reproductive organs. Sagittal section of pelvis showing placement of male reproductive organs.

Field Notes

Nudity

Before we move on to the reproductive system, I should tell you something about nudity. You have to look at naked bodies—fully naked breasts and genitals—to study human anatomy. Even more importantly, most anatomy and physiology (A&P) students move along into professions that require them to look at naked bodies. Breasts and genitals, even. You simply can't completely and practically know the body—or treat the body—without such exposure.

The problem with this is that our culture often tells us that looking at nakedness—especially the external reproductive organs and breasts—is not nice and even wrong. We can't avoid it by simply changing our minds—it's ingrained in our culture, which is a very powerful force that affects the development of our attitudes and beliefs. Because of this, it can also be very distracting.

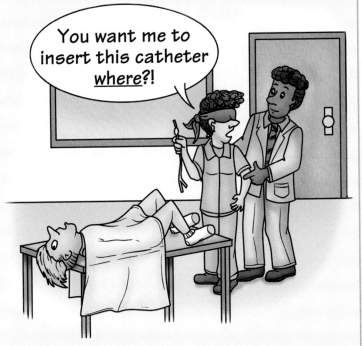

It's good to be aware of this cultural view as you begin your study of the reproductive system and have to look at genitals and breasts—or at least pictures of them. It's also good to be aware of this as you prepare for a profession in which you'll probably see far more breasts and genitals than you care to. Keep in mind that we all experience

Continued on page 293

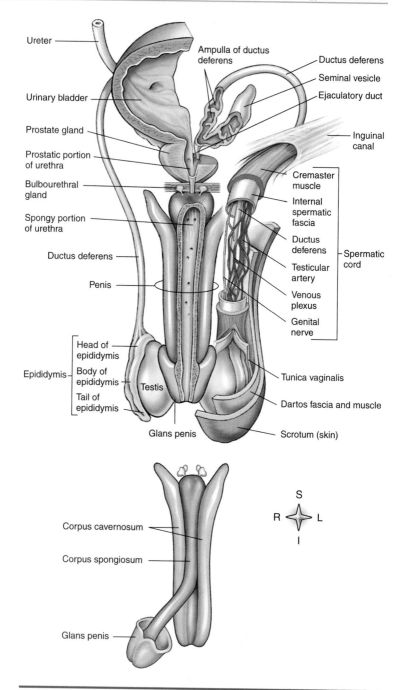

Figure 6-2 Anterior view of the male reproductive system. Illustration shows the testes, epididymis, ductus deferens, and glands of the male reproductive system in an isolation/dissection format.

Field Notes—cont'd

this built-in attitude (some more than others, of course), but we learn through time and experience to put it aside. Fortunately, cultural beliefs involving nakedness generally don't apply to anatomy classes or healing professions. However, nudity does take some getting used to for most people.

It's also good to be aware of this attitude when we do eventually deal with clients and colleagues—so that we can be sensitive to their possible attitudes and beliefs.

The same goes for terminology, too. If you can't say "penis" or "vagina" without giggling, then you had better find some way to overcome that before your A&P lab class—and certainly before your first clinical assignment. In addition, once you do get comfortable with the terms, then you should cultivate sensitivity in dealing with others nearby who haven't reached the same comfort level.

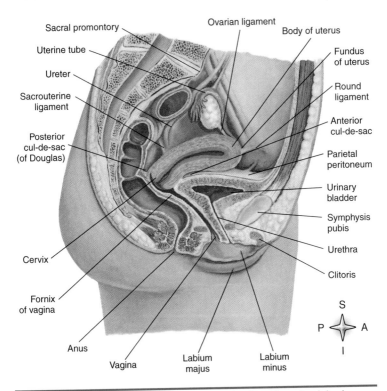

Figure 6-3 Female reproductive organs. Sagittal section of pelvis shows location of female reproductive organs.

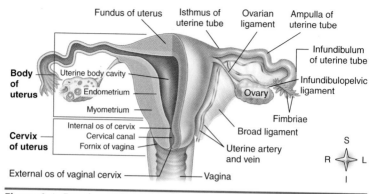

Figure 6-4 Female pelvic organs. Drawn in a partial frontal section, interior and exterior features of female reproductive organs of the pelvis are visible.

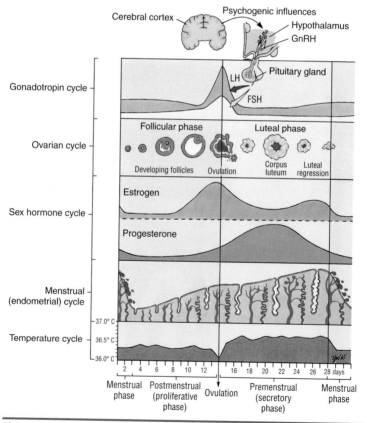

Figure 6-5 Female reproductive cycles. This diagram illustrates the interrelationships among the cerebral, hypothalamic, pituitary, ovarian, and uterine functions throughout a standard 28-day menstrual cycle. The variations in basal body temperature are also illustrated.

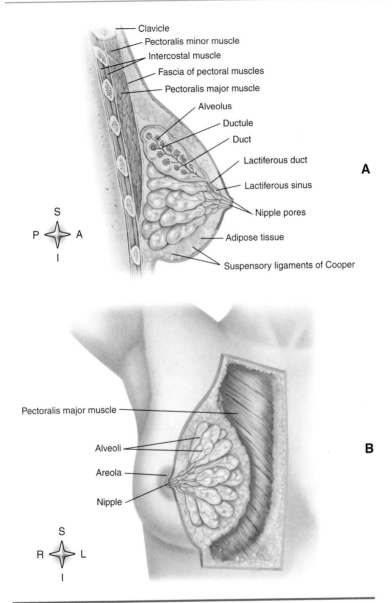

Clavicle
Pectoralis minor muscle
Intercostal muscle
Fascia of pectoral muscles
Pectoralis major muscle
Alveolus
Ductule
Duct
Lactiferous duct
Lactiferous sinus
Nipple pores
Adipose tissue
Suspensory ligaments of Cooper

A

S
P ← → A
I

Pectoralis major muscle
Alveoli
Areola
Nipple

B

S
R ← → L
I

Figure 6-6 The female breast. A, Sagittal section of a lactating breast. Notice how the glandular structures are anchored to the overlying skin and to the pectoral muscles by the suspensory ligaments of Cooper. Each lobule of glandular tissue is drained by a lactiferous duct that eventually opens through the nipple. **B,** Anterior view of a lactating breast. Overlying skin and connective tissue has been removed from the medial side to show the internal structure of the breast and underlying skeletal muscle. In non-lactating breasts, the glandular tissue is much less prominent, with adipose tissue comprising most of each breast.

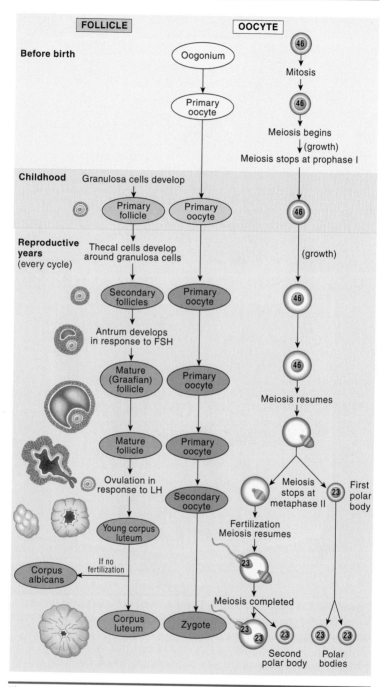

Figure 6-7 Oogenesis. Production of a mature ovum (oocyte) and subsequent fertilization are shown on the right as a series of cell divisions and on the left as a series of changes in the ovarian follicle.

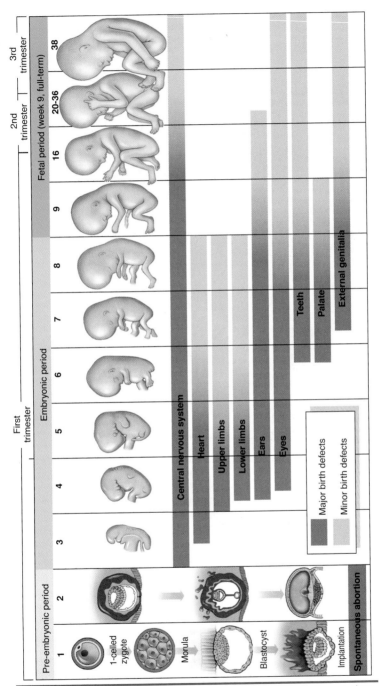

Figure 6-8 Critical periods of neonatal development. The red areas show when teratogens are most likely to cause major birth defects, and the yellow areas show when minor defects are more likely to arise.

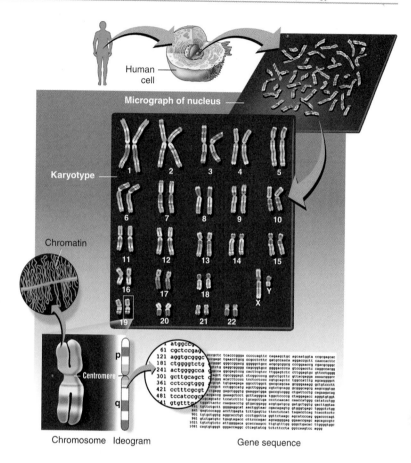

Human cell

Micrograph of nucleus

Karyotype

Chromatin

Centromere

p

q

Chromosome   Ideogram

Gene sequence

Figure 6-9 Human genome. A cell taken from the body is stained and photographed. A photograph of nuclear chromosomes is then cut and pasted, arranging each of the 46 chromosomes into numbered pairs of decreasing size to form a chart called the karyotype. Each chromosome is a coiled mass of chromatin (deoxyribonucleic acid [DNA]). In this figure, differentially stained bands in each chromosome appear as different, bright colors. Such bands are useful as reference points when identifying the locations of specific genes within a chromosome. The staining bands are also represented on an ideogram, or simple graph, of the chromosome as reference points to locate specific genes. The genes themselves are usually represented as the actual sequence of nucleotide bases, abbreviated at *a, c, g,* and *t.* In this figure, the sequence of one exon *(segment)* of a gene called GPI from chromosome 19 is shown. Each of these representations can be thought of as a type of "genetic map."

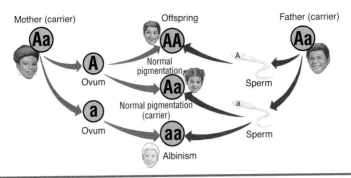

Figure 6-10 Inheritance of a recessive trait. Albinism is a recessive trait, producing abnormalities only in those with two recessive genes *(a)*. Presence of the dominant gene *(A)* prevents albinism.

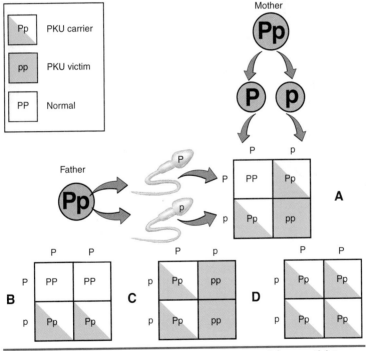

Figure 6-11 Punnett square. The Punnett square, named for geneticist Reginald Punnett, is a grid used to determine relative probabilities of producing offspring with specific gene combinations. Phenylketonuria (PKU) is a recessive disorder caused by the gene p. *P* is the normal gene. **A,** Possible results of cross between two PKU carriers. Because one in four of the offspring represented in the grid have PKU, a genetic counselor would predict a 25% chance that this couple will produce a PKU baby at each birth. **B,** Cross between a PKU carrier and a normal noncarrier. **C,** Cross between a PKU victim and a PKU carrier. **D,** Cross between a PKU victim and a normal noncarrier.